The Cancer Club

Stories From Past and Present Members of the Club No One Asks to Join

Nicola Wood

The Cancer Club
Stories From Past and Present Members of the Club No One Asks to Join
First published in Great Britain in 2025 by Inspired By Publishing

Cover design by: Inspired By Publishing

Photography by: Lisa McCormick Photography

ISBN: 9781068571206 Paperback

Published by: Inspired By Publishing

Dedication

For Steve and Gabriel – you are the reason this book exists and my inspiration for making it happen. My constant cheerleaders, hand-holders, and huggers.

For Caroline, Suzanne and Carmel, who have walked this path with me, and who just "got it." My heart aches that you can't read this but you've given me the determination to see it through and I hope you will be proud. You are dearly missed.

Acknowledgements

To my wonderful family and friends, thank you for standing by me, even when I'm being a proper stroppy cow. Your love, patience, and endless support have carried me through some dark days. I truly couldn't have done this without you. You kept me grounded, lifted me up, and believed in me when I couldn't believe in myself. I am eternally grateful.

To Steve, my incredible husband and greatest cheerleader, thank you for always reminding me "I can." You push me to be the best version of myself, never faltering, never complaining even when my work pulls me in a million directions. You've held our family together with strength and love, always protecting me and giving me the courage to chase my dreams. I love you more than words can say.

Gabriel, my little (well, taller than me now) ray of sunshine, your light has always broken through the cloudy days. Your smile, your energy and let's face it, your world-class hugs, well, they saved me more times than you'll ever know. You make me proud every single day, and you are my reason, my "Why." I hope you always believe that anything is possible, because it truly is. Have I told you today that I love you?

To my sister, Michelle, and my brother, Stephen, you have been my pillars, my constants, always ready to listen to my ridiculous emotional outbursts, calm me down, and remind me who I am. I couldn't have asked for better siblings, and I love you both dearly.

A special thanks to my NHS dream team – Mr. Clark, Miss Bromley, Caroline Buchanon and Caroline Tweedy – you saved my life. You guided me seamlessly through the toughest journey I've ever faced with such care, wisdom and patience, always answering my endless questions (even now). I'm so grateful for your expertise and compassion. You are my heroes.

Karen Verrill at Maggie's. I don't even know where to begin. Your support, knowledge and unwavering dedication to our local people is incredible. You are such a credit to our Northeast community and I thank my lucky stars for you.

Kirsty Wright, Marie Herron and Louise Hunter – nurses, clients, friends. You were there for me when I needed you the most and you have supported every crazy idea I've ever had. Thank you for believing in me and standing by my side.

Trevor Sorbie and the New Hair Team, you gave me my first step into the world of hair-loss solutions. Your training and guidance laid the foundation for what has become my life's mission. Thank you for helping me see that I was on the right path.

To our incredible clients, you are our inspiration. You come to us in your most vulnerable moments and your strength, resilience and raw honesty are what has become my life's mission. Thank you for trusting us with your journey.

To my brilliant work colleagues and work family, you are angels in every sense of the word. Beverley Mason, Alistair Nelson, Karen Young, Jemma Snowball, Janet Doyle, Caitlin Scarletts, Ellie Forbes, Kate Gaffney, Lorraine Vasey, Sarah Lewis, Niamh Geddes, Annabelle Lawson, Michelle Watson, Emma Tate, Caroline O'Sullivan and Rebecca Stoddart – your dedication, love and empathy are boundless and I am beyond grateful to have you by my side. You are the heart and soul of this mission and I don't tell you enough how truly amazing you all are. Thank you from the bottom of my heart.

Finally, to the brave contributors of this book, without you, none of this would be possible. Your stories, your honesty, your courage, it is all here, woven into these pages, touching lives and inspiring change. Thank you for trusting me with your experiences, for your wisdom, humour and tenacity. Together, we are creating something truly special. Thank you for being part of this journey with me.

Foreword

When I first met Nicola, it was instantly clear she's a woman with a deep sense of passion and purpose. Her story, like so many of the brave individuals I've had the pleasure to meet, is one of resilience, vision, and determination to turn her personal challenges into something that helps others.

Nicola's journey through breast cancer and autoimmune illness could have remained a personal battle. But instead, she turned it into something much larger than herself. She saw a gap in the support for women facing hair loss and she knew she could do better. Not just for herself, but for thousands of others in need. Through The Wonderful Wig Company, Nicola has changed lives. More than 15,000 people have stepped through her doors, finding not just wigs, but dignity, confidence and a genuine sense of care. Her mission to create safe, welcoming, and truly bespoke hair-loss services resonates and aligns deeply with my own values and everything I stand for: empowering individuals, breaking down barriers, and elevating the standards of care and inclusion. Nicola didn't stop there; her work to create the Inclusion Hair Network exemplifies her commitment to all communities, including minority and LGBTQIA+ groups. This is not just about hair, it's about creating spaces where everyone, no matter their background or circumstance, feels seen, understood, and supported.

Nicola's story is a powerful reminder of the difference one person can make, even in life's most challenging moments. As you read this book, you'll not only learn about her personal triumph over adversity, but you'll also see how she's used that strength to inspire and uplift others. She has taken her experiences and used them as a driving force for good, revolutionising how women facing hair loss are treated both medically and emotionally. I'm honoured to write this foreword and to celebrate Nicola's remarkable achievements. Her courage, generosity, and unwavering commitment to supporting others is a shining example of the power of compassion. I know her story will move and inspire everyone who reads it.

Simone Roche MBE
CEO & Founder, We Are Power
Honorary Captain, Royal Navy

Preface

This book has been thoughtfully crafted to accompany you on your journey with cancer, whether you've received a diagnosis yourself or are supporting someone who has. You'll likely find stories that resonate deeply, some that lift your spirits, others that bring tears, and a few that may catch you by surprise. The power of human resilience continues to astound me. When you need support, comfort, or a reminder that you're not walking this path alone, I hope this book offers you strength. Each chapter is like a gentle hug, a reminder that you are brave, loved, and supported by a community that stands with you.

Bringing this book to life didn't come from a single moment of clarity; it feels like something I've always known would happen. Meeting countless individuals touched by cancer, I realised the weight of responsibility to gather and share their stories. The glimpses of experience in these pages reflect only a fraction of how cancer changes lives. Each story is unique, shaped by personal diagnosis, treatments, and the profound journey of living with cancer.

I hope that within these stories, you find comfort, hope, and inspiration. I've also included a selection of resources that may provide valuable support. During challenging times, it can be overwhelming to know where to turn or who to trust, especially when the noise of social media and online communities becomes too much. The resources shared here are either personally used by me or recommended by others in the book so you can trust their reliability. Some stories may be hard to read, and while I wish I could paint cancer as all rainbows and sunshine, we know that's not the reality. These accounts are shared with sensitivity and honesty, aiming to offer solace no matter the outcome.

Feel free to use the QR code below to access the resources we've compiled for your journey.

Contents

Introduction
Welcome to the Ride

It was a typical Saturday night; I was excited to have some fun as I got all dolled up for a proper fancy charity event with the girls at a local rugby club. I had a beautiful, long, sequin-covered golden dress – I couldn't wait to wear it. But first, the inevitable shimmy into my Spanx!

There I was squashing and squeezing, not very majestically, into this shapewear set that looked more like it was a baby's washed-out onesie. The unglamorous task of getting myself into this torturous thing was underway, starting with one leg and then another. Stuffing the usual skin, lumps, and bumps into the one-piece – finally getting to my boobs. One big inhale and in went my left boob, and then I braced myself. As anybody who has tried this will confirm, getting the second breast in is more challenging because it's what brings it all "together."

A big inhale and I went for it; as I did, I remember thinking, "Oh, what was **that**?" I had noticed a tiny lump against the back wall of my chest, unlike all the other lumps I had just squeezed into my Spanx. It was tiny, it was very small, but it was most definitely a lump. By the time I had completed contorting my body and covering the sensational under-armour, I was content knowing I would have a great night and reminded myself to come back to this lump tomorrow.

I had a great night (as far as I can remember). I had gone out, looking gorgeous with very little thought to what I had just discovered. However, that little lump was my first sign.

Unknowingly, at that moment, I had joined the **CANCER CLUB**.

Without warning. Without consent. Without a choice.

My name is Nicola Wood, and I was diagnosed with breast cancer at 36 years old. I had a husband, a son, family, friends, and a successful business. Now, I have all of those – and so much more.

If you're reading this book then it's likely you're on a similar path as me, and if you're somewhere at the beginning of your journey, I can only imagine what's going on in your mind right now. Even as someone who's been through it, I can't tell you what will happen for sure. This won't be the book for that – if such a book even exists, please, tell me where to find it. What I can tell you is that you will amaze yourself in the most wondrous ways in the months to come. And whatever happens, own your journey and embrace it.

I can honestly say that my life has changed for the better since my diagnosis. I believe I was meant to get cancer; otherwise, I would never have been forced off the hamster wheel of life. I wouldn't have learned to stop constantly wanting more, nor would I have achieved what I was truly meant to. I know how incredibly fortunate I am to be able to say this, and I hope this book helps you feel the same.

How can I be so sure? Thanks to my journey with cancer, I have had the opportunity to advocate for others and impact the lives of others with similar diagnoses, and I have crossed paths with more than 15,000 extraordinary individuals who have shown me how capable we are of unwavering resilience, determination, strength and our ability to turn painful events into something wonderful.

The people I've met are the reason you have this book in your hands today. As you'll notice from my style, I'm no seasoned author, which was at the heart of my decision to put the book together. It was important to me to write a book for normal people, by normal people.

Nobody who has contributed to this book is a professional writer. Yet because we care so passionately about helping you to have a more positive experience through your cancer, we have each written our stories from our hearts. They are real, they are raw and they are offered to support you to make sense of it all in a way that helps you to think, "Yes, me too."

When you first start hearing and talking about cancer, it feels like learning a foreign language. The jargon and phrases are confusing until you're fully immersed in it and have no choice but to understand. Cancer can be the loneliest place on Earth. Even if you're surrounded by family and friends, or are the most popular person around, you're still alone with your cancer.

Cancer is a life event that affects more than half the world, and it brings much more than just trauma. The more we talk about it, the more people will understand, and the less frightening it will seem. By breaking it down and having open, honest conversations, maybe it won't feel as terrifying.

What if "cancer" wasn't such a frightening word? What if it wasn't such a taboo subject? What if people diagnosed with cancer were more visible on TV and online?

With greater awareness of cancer and the importance of early diagnosis, we could save many more lives, rather than letting the assumption that cancer equals a death sentence persist. People might not put off going for mammograms, smears and general health checks; they might take it seriously and embrace it as a positive self-care thing to do for themselves. Anything that allows people to understand cancer better, however little, is a good thing.

This book is for anybody with cancer. It's also for anybody who is supporting someone with cancer. I believe that we all have a responsibility to know how cancer affects people, how we support them to navigate their cancer, be able to say the "right" things, and understand what they may need and how they might be feeling. I hope that you'll find at least one story, or a golden nugget of wisdom or inspiration, in these pages that helps you realise you've got this. You are not alone.

What you're about to read is a collection of stories, reflections, anecdotes, thoughts, and lessons that helped me get through my journey and will, hopefully, help you through yours. Let this be a source of companionship with a sprinkling of wisdom. Instead of viewing this as a book of advice – I'm sure you've heard more than enough on a situation that can't be changed – think of it like relaxing with a cup of tea, having a chat with patients, carers, friends, family, doctors, nurses, and everyday people, just like you and me.

Take comfort as you hear the words of those people who like you are navigating the unknown scary roller coaster of cancer. Hear their voices as their words come alive on the pages, wrapping their arms around you to comfort and guide you.

Chapter 1
Strength and Surrender

The morning after the rugby charity event, I was lying in bed feeling worse for wear and recounting the night to my husband, now free of the sequined frock and torturous body stocking. As I went through the evening, moment by moment, I suddenly remembered, "Actually, Steve, whilst I was getting ready, I thought I felt a tiny lump in my breast. Let me see if I can find it and I'll show you what I mean."

Steve gently touched where I had noticed the lump and confirmed, "I can feel something, Nicola, but you know, boobs can be lumpy. I'm sure it's nothing," he said, offering me some comfort. "But you should go to the doctor and have it checked."

I didn't go to the doctor.

I waited a few more weeks, not giving it much thought – nothing more than a little niggle at the back of my mind. Finally, I decided to make an appointment with my doctor. I even recall feeling a little stupid for wasting their time. It was merely a job that I was looking to check off my never-ending to-do list.

I was familiar with my doctors and the team I was seeing, having been diagnosed with rheumatoid arthritis in my 20s. So, on my one day off, I rushed in without a moment to spare. I was a busy mam – that's "mum" for you outside of the Northeast – with a business that doesn't run itself. My doctor did a quick examination, confirmed there was a lump, and told me he'd have to refer me to the breast clinic. I left the doctor's surgery and got on with my day, no major alarm bells ringing.

The next day, a call came from the doctor's office to book me into the Queen Elizabeth Symptomatic Breast Clinic with my referral date. I didn't completely understand at the time, but this clinic is for anyone with symptoms of breast cancer, a brilliant service and a one-stop shop. "Great, I can rule this lump out and get on with my life," I thought to myself.

On the day of my appointment, I went to Queen Elizabeth by myself. I had told my husband I was going but I wouldn't let him come with me because I'm that bloody independent. It's quite irritating to everyone around me. I met Dr. Clark, who confirmed that he could feel the lump but wasn't overly concerned. There would be some tests to go through, and he would see me again at the end of them.

My first mammogram was a very strange experience indeed. For the unfamiliar, it's essentially an X-ray where your boobs are contorted and squeezed between two pieces of plastic to check for anything out of the ordinary. It felt weird and unexpectedly uncomfortable, and I've been in some uncomfortably contorted situations, as you know. I couldn't help but wonder how they accommodated all shapes and sizes of breasts!

As I sat in the waiting room with other women, all of whom looked terrified and were taking it much more seriously than I was, I recall thinking, "I'm one of the youngest here." Then, rather foolishly in retrospect, I thought, "Wow, some of these people have cancer," as I noticed their bald heads. I believed I was going through routine procedures; there was no possibility of cancer, especially when Dr. Clark told me at the end of the appointment that he was fairly convinced it was simply a fibroadenoma, a growth of sorts. After a CT scan and breast biopsies were taken, I left feeling reassured, with a leaflet about fibroadenomas tucked safely in my bag.

I can honestly say that I did not give it another thought. I completely forgot about the tests, the lump, and everything else. I went back to regular life. I hadn't even told my siblings about the lump at that point. I was so used to going to the hospital for tests and treatment for my arthritis that I took it all in my stride. At the time, I didn't know enough about cancer or the associated jargon to understand the reality of the tests.

Two weeks later, I received a telephone call from an unknown number. It was Caroline, the kind nurse who had taken me under her wing when I first went to Queen Elizabeth. "Nic, we've got the results from your tests. We need you to come back in so we can discuss them," she said.

"I can't come in. I'm working with clients and won't be able to make it for a couple of weeks. Can't you tell me over the phone? Dr. Clark told me it was a fibroadenoma, so there was nothing to worry about. You can give me that news on the phone." I replied.

"Sorry, Nicola, we must deliver all results face-to-face, regardless of what they are. I need you to come in," Caroline insisted, reluctant to take no for an answer.

So, I agreed.

I was naive.

I was dismissive.

I was ticking another job off my to-do list.

In my usual last-minute style, I bounded through the doors of the Queen Elizabeth on the day of my appointment, running late. I rushed through the corridors, getting lost in the maze of coloured zones as I tried to find my way to the breast care department. When I finally reached the waiting room, I was once again surrounded by older women and their companions. Steve had offered to accompany me, but I had firmly declined. I had squeezed this appointment between 27 other things I had on my list; I didn't need anyone with me for this. I assumed everyone else in the room had it much worse. I believed I would be given the all-clear and be on my way.

I was pleasantly surprised when the friendly face of Caroline opened the double doors and called my name. Striding behind her, the doors swung shut, and suddenly a wave of fear washed over me. I think often about that moment; in that split second, I knew, with every fibre of my being – **I knew!** In the consultation room sat another nurse and my consultant. There was a shift, something had changed. Dr. Clark began to talk, affirming what I knew. I heard the words fall from his mouth, "I'm sorry, Nicola, I got it wrong. It wasn't a fibroadenoma. You have breast cancer."

"Reality check, Nicola. You f*cking idiot," I thought. I was so angry with myself.

Over the next few minutes, Dr. Clark, holding my hand, calmly explained what I needed to know – the type of cancer, the size of the tumour, and the suggested treatment. I was in shock. All I heard was *cancer*.

The rest of the appointment blurred into a haze of hysterical emotions. They wanted to call Steve, but I insisted they didn't. My mind was racing, trying to grasp what this all meant. No way could Steve hear this over the phone.

They moved me to a quiet room to help me gather my thoughts and prepare for the drive home. Someone brought tea, tea always helps. "Pull yourself together, Nicola" - these were the loudest words in my head, my age-old response to any crisis.

I sat in my car for what felt like hours, trying to make sense of it all. I asked myself who I should call first, my sister Michelle or Steve. They were the only ones who knew I was at the hospital. In my head, I spiralled into catastrophe. I was convinced I was dying. It felt like the end. I was convinced the consultant had made a mistake - it wouldn't be the first time. They were initially so reassuring that it wasn't cancer and there I was sat in the car, feeling like I was staring death in the face. Cancer = death. That's all there was to it.

All the practical worries started flooding in: Would Steve have enough money to care for our son Gabe alone? What would happen to my business? How would I pay the bills if I couldn't work? Sh*t, what if Gabe doesn't remember me? Would Steve replace me if I die? More than anything, I was consumed with thoughts of Gabe. My baby. What would he do without his mammy? It felt like my insides were being ripped apart. I even started thinking I'd have to write a manual for Steve on how to care for Gabe.

Every second dragged on. Part of me wanted to stay in that car forever, hoping I'd wake up and find out this was all a nightmare. Eventually, I pulled myself together enough to call Steve and see if he was home, forcing a cheerful voice so he wouldn't sense how broken I felt. Then I called my sister and asked her to come by, making up some trivial excuse just so I could tell her in person.

When Steve saw me, he didn't need to ask. He just held me as I broke down, trying to piece together enough words to explain. My sister arrived soon after, and while I was in the middle of a meltdown, she calmly started making sense of the situation. She shifted into "doer" mode, reassuring me that I didn't have to worry about telling anyone else right now, that would be her job. She'd handle it all while I tried to hold on through the storm.

The next few days and weeks were probably the most horrendous moments of my life. I have nothing to compare those feelings to, except perhaps the grief you feel when someone dies and you're utterly distraught for a time.

And in a way, there had been a death. Not in the biological sense that everyone associates with cancer, but in the sense that the Nicola who walked into the Queen Elizabeth Hospital that day was gone.

I would never be her again.

Digesting a cancer diagnosis is not an overnight job. It's like a hand grenade has been thrown from nowhere directly into the middle of your life. Everything you've known and assumed blows up in your face. Blow after blow, shifts and changes arrive. For me, it was an incredibly long and winding process of letting things go and learning to navigate the fear and anger at each new stage. I had to learn and master acceptance, over the many years to come.

I decided to initially only share the diagnosis with my husband, family, and siblings, Michelle and Stephen. The doctor had suggested it was in an early stage and curable, but nothing was sure until more test results, so I decided I would work right up until the day before my surgery then I would have to be off-the-radar during my months-long recovery.

Steve and I carefully considered how we would tell Gabriel, trusting that we could do it in a way that would help him understand and be part of what was going on. We sat down with him, took a deep breath, and explained as much as we could in a way that he could process at the age of six. It was our number one priority to normalise this for him.

The thought of having to tell other people outside of my family - especially my clients - that I had cancer was gut-wrenching. I couldn't face the thought of endless conversations seeing their heads tilt, their faces full of pity and naturally wanting to offer me their sympathy. As an extroverted hairdresser, I loved the joyful and fun conversations I had with my clients as I looked at them in the mirror. I often felt like their therapist, coach and best friend wrapped into one! Now they'd want to turn the table and be that for me. It filled me with utter dread.

As any hairdresser will tell you, news travels fast in our industry and it was playing on my mind that my clients would notice I was not at work for several months. I didn't want my then-six-year-old son to hear anything from other mams while at the playground, so I made a decision. I took control of my fears and sent out an email letting all my clients know.

I also wanted to take control of my story. I set the record straight and let people know I didn't have a life-limiting illness. It was likely I'd be gone for a few months, yes, but I would soon be back to normal. My plan worked across my close network. I chose to boldly ignore anyone who, after 20 years of silence, tried to re-enter my life with intrusive emails just because they heard through the grapevine about my cancer.

Humans are so accessible these days. People can write and they can ring. They can text. They can Whatsapp, they can Facebook, they can Instagram, they can Snapchat. And everyone means so well. But you can only say the same thing so many times, over and over again. "I'm fine," "We're waiting on test results," "I don't have any more news," "No, thank you. There's nothing I need." I didn't want to sound ungrateful, but I knew it was time to set boundaries.

I sent one last message to all my channels saying I needed some time to completely disengage and switch off. If anybody needed me, they could get to me via my husband or my sister. In doing this, anybody who didn't have their numbers disappeared from my radar and I could stop worrying about upsetting or offending them and concentrate on what mattered most to me.

Those who mattered were my little family at home, and the energetic six-year-old waiting for me to come and play. I did everything I could to be a normal mam; a mam who wasn't going to die, a mam who could still laugh and chase, who read bedtime stories and hugged tightly while sharing our wishes for sweet dreams each night. My son was and still is my everything, and I wanted his world to keep shining bright. I didn't want him to be afraid of cancer.

One of the hardest things when you find out that you have cancer is sitting with that knowledge. This "thing" is inside you until you find out your treatment plan.

Waiting for more results, more scans, more tests, more blood tests, more needles. It feels endless. But the hardest part of all this for me was not the scan, not the appointment, not the needles, it was the waiting between. Never knowing if it might get worse, knowing that you have cancer, that it's in you and it's growing. All you can do is WAIT!

I was desperate to get the bloody plan. I'm a doer in life, so that feeling of idly waiting around and maybe losing time to stop the "thing" from growing was frustrating. Eventually, my plan was explained. I felt relief that the waiting was over, but knew it was only the next move in a long tactical game.

The surgery date couldn't come fast enough. I felt I was being slowly tortured once I knew when it was, as I counted down the days. I didn't care that someone was going to cut into my breast; surgery itself was not frightening to me, I needed to feel like I was moving forward, to feel like I was doing and not waiting.

Surgery day finally came. Waking up in the hospital with the knowledge that the cancer was gone felt like I had just won the lottery. It was such a relief to know it had been removed. But the feeling of elation did not last long. After the surgery, the nagging weight of the wait took hold again as we went on to the next steps. Radiotherapy was explained to me as a backup. It's a bit like an insurance policy against recurrence or spread. I was pleased to have a plan, and I was beginning to allow Steve and my inner circle to support me fully.

I have always been such an independent person. Letting Steve take the reins was uncomfortable but I knew I couldn't bear the weight alone. Our relationship had shifted the moment he learned I had cancer. I became this delicate little flower that needed looking after and protecting. Nobody would get near me. If you wanted to get to me, you needed to get through Steve. He wouldn't allow anyone to upset me. Everything would be everybody else's fault, never mine. I could've gotten away with murder with his help if I wanted to. Anything that needed doing, he did. Anything I wanted he said yes to, although I'm still waiting for my teacup Yorkshire Terrier!

I could see his pain and his grief for the loss of our future, the one we dreamt about and planned together. He was also in pain and reeling from the shock. Neither of us knew what the future held. Steve tried not to show his worry around me. I struggle to imagine our roles being reversed and how I would feel being unable to take away his pain or worry. I do not underestimate how hard it was for him to watch me suffer at this time and to keep putting on a brave face, endlessly trying to lift my spirits, give me hope, and maintain positivity.

While my husband became an action-man, my siblings became my emotional base. I can be intense when it comes to my emotions, so thankfully, I have a sister and brother who are used to my outbursts – even more so during my cancer journey. Steve would do all the practical stuff, throwing himself into the "doing" part of things: the appointments, the heavy lifting, and anything else that I wanted. Meanwhile, Michelle and Stephen would support me by talking about my feelings and the future.

The thing is, when you are with those you love and you know they are crippled by your news, you want to shield them too. You don't want to say just how scared you are because you know they're also scared. My siblings and my husband accepted my screaming and my endless tears. They accepted all of me, so however I turned up on any day was just fine.

Acceptance plays a big role in going through cancer and its aftermath. Accepting how you feel in the moment, accepting the changes in your body, and accepting that it's okay to feel a range of emotions. Embracing this acceptance allows you to move forward with grace and resilience, knowing that it's okay to feel all that you are feeling.

The stories in the following section all touch on coming to terms with vulnerability and loss of control after a cancer diagnosis while learning how to balance your pre-cancer identity with the reality of treatment and emotional adjustment. They delve into the psychological journey of feeling as if your identity and independence are being taken over by the illness and the need to regain a sense of control over your life. I invite you to read and listen to the different journeys below that tackle the path you may now be on.

1

Learning to Accept the Unexpected

By Lauren Sharp

After a cancer diagnosis, everything changes. It forces you to re-evaluate your life, what matters, and where your priorities lie. For me, that realisation came on 8 May 2021, when I found a lump in my right breast.

At first, I wasn't too alarmed. Cancer didn't run in my family, and everyone assured me that most lumps like this were harmless. I didn't think of myself as someone who would get cancer but I still went straight to the doctor to have it checked.

Following an urgent referral and a private health assessment, my initial ultrasound came back clear, which reassured me. However, additional core samples revealed the worst: on 17 May 2022, I was diagnosed with oestrogen-receptive breast cancer at 34 years old.

Although it was Stage 1 and hadn't spread, the doctor emphasised the cancer's high grade, meaning it could be aggressive. I was in complete shock. I sat in the small room thinking, "F*ck," as reality began to set in. I wasn't ready to grasp the enormity of what was happening. I thought, "It's just a touch of cancer, they'll operate, and I'll be back at work next week." I was in denial.

Surgery was scheduled quickly. A mastectomy, immediate reconstruction, IVF preservation, chemotherapy, and more surgeries followed all within four months. Then, in January 2023, genetic tests showed I had the CHEK-2 mutation, prompting a preventative mastectomy of my left breast. Unfortunately, complications meant further surgeries to remove the implant. Despite all this, my incredible breast team at Durham Hospital never gave up on me.

Throughout treatment, I kept convincing myself I didn't really have cancer, it was just a touch of it. I tried to stick to my routines, pushing myself to keep life as normal as possible for my daughter, Isla, who was only three. But as my condition worsened, I could no longer pretend. Stress consumed me, sleepless nights became routine and I withdrew from everything.

Losing my hair was the turning point. I could no longer hide what was happening. I hated missing out on moments with Isla: nursery performances, birthday parties, and even simple trips to the park. I felt disconnected and overwhelmed with worry, making it hard to stay present.

Through it all, my husband James was my rock. He attended every appointment, helped with my medication, and brought endless M&S supplies. He patiently listened to my fears, always staying calm and reassuring, even when I lost my hair. After shaving my head, he told me, "You look great, a new style for you," while I cried. His support kept me going and focused on staying strong and healthy.

Acknowledging That I Had Cancer

For a long time, I told myself that I didn't really have cancer and that it wasn't a big deal. I avoided talking about it, but eventually, the emotional toll caught up to me. I realised I needed to face the truth and open up about my experience.

Attending support groups was challenging at first, as I didn't feel like anyone my age could relate. But slowly, I found ways to cope and focus on what I could control.

What Helped Me

Routine. I realised that hiding under the covers wasn't going to help. Establishing a routine gave me a sense of control and kept me grounded.

Exercise. Walking in nature helped me clear my mind and strengthen my body. At first, I could only walk for a few minutes, but gradually, I built up my stamina.

Therapy. Talking to a therapist gave me the space to process my emotions. It wasn't an instant fix, but it helped me understand that emotional recovery is a long journey.

Wigs. Wearing a wig allowed me to reclaim a sense of normality. I didn't have to start every conversation with an explanation of my condition, and it helped me feel more in control of my appearance.

Moving Forward

My advice for anyone facing a cancer diagnosis is to keep moving forward, even if it's just one small step at a time. Be yourself, maybe an even braver version of yourself. Do what makes you happy and don't let cancer define who you are or where your life is headed.

Now, I feel stronger than ever. I want to help others who, like me, struggle to find support as young women facing cancer. My journey has been hard, but if sharing my story helps others realise their strength, it will have been worth it.

2

Embracing the New You

By Marie Herring

My breast cancer diagnosis came from a routine mammogram. At first, I felt lucky it was caught early, and the doctors seemed hopeful it was just a benign cyst. But with every step, the news got worse. A biopsy confirmed it was cancer, and while I held onto hope that a lumpectomy and radiotherapy would be enough, the discovery of cancer in three out of four lymph nodes meant I'd need chemotherapy too.

With my medical background, I had an idea of the potential treatments and risks. My attitude was, "Let's just get on with it," but for my husband, Phil, it was much harder. He felt helpless and became overprotective. To manage his worries, we created a "worry monster" named Philomena. He'd write down his fears and feed them to the monster, a small but effective way to cope.

My best friend was my constant support both to me and Phil. She acted as my advocate through the confusing maze of treatment options and supported me during the hardest moments.

I navigated the overwhelming flood of information and decisions, including which medical trials to join. I chose to participate in a trial that offered extra protection post-treatment but declined one that seemed too uncertain.

Following surgery, which I recovered well from, I underwent six rounds of chemotherapy and 20 doses of radiotherapy. The trial was also to take medication to prevent the complications of heart disease post-treatment.

Knowing that hair loss was inevitable, I decided to take control of my appearance. I had my eyebrows tattooed to keep a sense of normality and maintain some glamour. Finding someone willing to do it so close to my treatment was difficult, but I was determined. I clung to my usual look as a way of maintaining control during a time when so much felt out of my hands.

I'm quite a private person and did not want sympathy. If my colleagues were not part of my social life before my diagnosis, I didn't need them now. Some may think I became insular, but I didn't have time for superficial politeness. I didn't need passengers on my journey, I needed the sincerity and honesty of my close family and friends.

I tried where possible to maintain my life but when I was not feeling so good I would often go off the grid and the people who knew me well accepted this.

Facing Hair Loss

During my first course of treatment, I was quite obsessive in documenting when I was well and when I wasn't. This was because I knew treatment would become progressively more difficult and I still wanted to enjoy a normal life when I felt well. Life became very planned and structured.

As my treatment progressed, my energy waned, and I could only manage four out of the six chemotherapy sessions before being hospitalised twice. I hated being in the hospital and fought to go home as soon as I could.

I knew hair loss was coming, so I prepared. My hairdresser had recently opened The Wonderful Wig Company, and she understood exactly what I needed: the balance between maintaining my appearance and feeling like myself. We planned to cut my hair once it started to fall out, which it did around Christmas. Clumps came away as I ran my hands through it.

Though I was ready for it, nothing prepares you for how others treat you differently when you look sick. The stares, and the sympathy, made me feel like I was carrying a sign that said, "I have cancer." At home, I didn't wear a wig or hat, but when I answered the door without one, the shocked looks reminded me of my illness.

One day at Seaham Beach, I slipped on a muddy path and lost my hat. People rushed to help as soon as they saw my bald head. I quickly put the hat back on and carried on walking as if nothing had happened, trying to reclaim some sense of normality.

Embracing Change

Going to the hairdresser with my best friend kept some sense of routine alive, even though my hair was gone. I'd take my wig in to be washed, and they'd treat it like any other head of hair. It was a comforting routine. At night, I wore a cotton hat because my bald head got cold, but the hardest part came when my hair began to grow back.

It was nothing like my old long, straight hair. Instead, it grew back grey and curly. Despite this, I felt liberated to finally shower and go. My hairdresser kept my spirits up, trimming my hair and helping me stay positive, even though it would take time before I could fully style it again.

Heading back to work with grey hair felt daunting. One colleague called me "brave" for not dyeing it as if I had a choice. Their lack of sensitivity shocked me, but I reminded myself that these small steps toward normality were victories.

Finding Strength

Through it all, I stayed focused on what mattered most: keeping control over my life, even in the smallest ways. I realised that getting up and dressed each day, no matter how hard, was an act of defiance against cancer. It was a reminder that I was still here, still fighting.

Looking back, I realise the importance of letting go of what no longer serves me. I focused on the people and routines that mattered, releasing anything that added unnecessary stress. While I don't see myself as a hero, I'm always willing to help others who face this journey. Cancer is a long-term condition, but it doesn't define me.

Advice for Others

Stay positive and document your chemotherapy cycles so you can plan around the days you feel well. Let go of anyone or anything that doesn't add value to your life. Cancer doesn't have to define you. Focus on managing your symptoms, but don't feel the need to be a hero.

My key takeaway: It's not over until the fat lady sings. And no news is good news.

3

Growing Up in the Face of Cancer

By Laura Meredith

I remember sitting on the stairs, listening to the hushed, grown-up conversation in the living room. My parents and step-sister were talking, mentioning words like "cancer" and "serious". I could hear the terror in their voices, using words that sent fear racing through me.

I couldn't believe it. I asked myself, isn't cancer something that only happens to old people? My mum, my world, couldn't have cancer. What if she dies? It felt impossible to wrap my head around.

Mum and I were inseparable; we spent all our time together since my dad worked long hours. Living in the middle of nowhere meant I had no friends to distract me from what was happening at home.

For days, I pretended I hadn't heard the conversation, but I knew the truth. When mum came home from her appointment, I hugged her tightly and simply said, "I know, it's okay, you're going to be fine, Mum." Inside, I had already made up my mind that I would do everything I could to support her through this.

Mum's ovarian cancer diagnosis came in 1999 after she experienced heavy periods, pain and poor appetite. What followed was a whirlwind of a full hysterectomy and chemotherapy.

The treatment seemed brutal at times, and just before mum's surgery, I was diagnosed with ME, and struggled to keep up with school. When the school found out about mum's illness, they arranged for home tutors, though it was hard to focus on studying when all I could think about was mum.

The operation was a success, but the toll on mum's body was clear. She tried to put on a brave face, but I could see her pain and fear. Telling someone it's going to be okay when you have no idea if it really will be - that's one of the hardest things I've ever had to do.

A Crash Course in Adulthood

Mum's six rounds of chemotherapy began, and we had no idea what to expect. My life changed overnight.

Suddenly, I had to grow up fast. I took on all the chores, learned to cook, and even mastered online shopping.

My tutors came a couple of days a week, but my real focus was running the house and making sure mum didn't have to worry about anything.

Whenever Mum felt well enough, family and friends would visit, and we'd try to go out and enjoy ourselves. But being a normal teenager wasn't much of an option. Mum did her best to take me to see my friends, but some days it felt like the walls were closing in.

Dad, being old-school, was all about stoic support, nods, handshakes, and stiff-upper-lip encouragement. Mum was the opposite, fiercely protective, like a lioness. We became each other's source of comfort during the darkest days.

Mum had her lows, days when she hit rock bottom, but I could never show weakness. I saved my tears for late at night when I was alone or walking the dog. Sometimes I wanted to scream, but I held it in, knowing that strength was needed for Mum.

The Little Things

Mum's chemo treatments were hard on her, especially when she began losing her hair. Each dose made it thinner and it started falling out. It was time for us to step in. Mum didn't want to go to a salon, so Dad offered to shave her head. I noticed how much he was struggling and I took over, chatting with Mum to keep things light.

We laughed together as we visited a wig specialist, choosing a style she liked. Nothing prepares you for the ups and downs of cancer, but we made it through that day together. We found a wig that Mum was happy with.

We were told the wig could only be washed by hand in cool water and shaken out before leaving to dry naturally. Joking and giggling all the way home, we imagined leaving the wig on the washing line and crows choosing it to build their nests in. There were the usual worries about the wig flying off in the wind or bending down and people noticing. With some practice and lots of reassurance, Mum became less self-conscious.

We kept a stock of lemon sorbet in the freezer for the days when Mum couldn't face food. The metallic taste in her mouth from chemo was awful, and the sorbet helped.

Comfort became a priority, soft blankets, fans, her favourite magazines and good slippers. These little things made all the difference.

On Mum's good weeks, we went to bingo nights with the neighbours and played board games like Scrabble. These moments helped us maintain a sense of normality, even when life was anything but normal.

Friends and family would often call on the telephone to see how Mum was doing. The same questions over and over again were utterly exhausting! I knew they all cared and meant well. My grandparents would call, every evening at 9pm, to check in and I loved receiving this call. The love they gave was magical.

Thank You, Mum

Sadly, after five years of fighting, Mum lost her battle with cancer. But she left me with strength, grit, and determination that I carry with me every day. Her bravery during treatment shaped the person I've become. She taught me to follow my dreams, to appreciate life, and to never take anything for granted.

Recently, we moved to a smallholding in Scotland, where we're planning to offer free holidays to families with a member undergoing cancer treatment. We want to provide them with a safe place to escape the daily grind of treatments, meet our animals, and just relax.

If you ever need to support someone with cancer, hold them tight. Tell them you love them every single day because tomorrow isn't promised. Laugh often, stay positive, and cherish every moment you have together.

4

Balancing Self and Support

By Marilyn Cook and Chloë Bisson

Marilyn:

My journey with cancer began at 52 when I asked my doctor why I hadn't been called for a mammogram. In Jersey, there's no automatic system like in the UK, but my doctor arranged one for me. It seemed like a routine check until a week later, I received a letter asking me to return for further tests. Although the team initially didn't seem too concerned, they referred me to Andy Borthwick-Clark, who noticed a shadow on my X-ray. He was adamant about further investigation, and for that, I'll always be grateful.

Chloë:

It was 2004, my 16th birthday. I was surrounded by friends and family at an Italian restaurant, everyone singing "Happy Birthday," but inside, I felt hollow. Something was missing. Mum wasn't there – she was in surgery having a cancerous lump removed. It was the first birthday I'd spent without her, and it felt wrong.

Marilyn:

In the operating room, the two surgeons inserted the wire to get to the exact spot where the shadow appeared on the X-ray. Here, they found cancer. They removed a golf-ball-sized piece of breast tissue. They decided, between the two of them, to do a bit of wizardry and move the flesh around, inside the breast, to fill the hole and then stitch it in place, so there was no dip, just a slightly smaller breast!

Chloë and I believe in the significance of dates and numbers, so when my operation fell on her birthday, we found some comfort in it. Despite the surgery's success, my absence on her special day weighed heavily on both of us.

Chloë:

Me and my mum have always been interested in spirituality - numbers and dates have always been important. Even though neither of us wanted her to have the operation on my birthday, we knew it was this date for a reason.

I left my birthday celebration early to visit Mum in the hospital. Being the only child of divorced parents, I was used to handling tough situations on my own, but walking into that hospital alone was one of the loneliest moments of my teenage years. Seeing Mum, though, brought immense relief.

Marilyn:

Five months after the operation, I travelled to Southampton for radiotherapy. During my stay, I realised I could help others by documenting my journey and taking pictures of the facilities, the staff, and even the local coffee shops. I wanted to provide a roadmap for other patients facing the same overwhelming experience.

Chloë would come and stay too and we would make it feel like a holiday; having fun, going for walks, ferry trips, shopping - we tried to make the most of the situation we found ourselves in. We have always had a strong bond but this experience made us realise how precious life is.

Chloë:

Being apart from my mum while she underwent treatment was tough. The uncertainty gnawed at me - how was she coping? Who was there to support her? But during this time, I learned how vital it was to care for my well-being too. Balancing my healing with supporting her became a lesson in resilience.

I recognised the importance of allowing myself time to heal. There was a charity called After Breast Cancer that supported us and paid for me to go and stay with her in Southampton.

Marilyn:

As I continued my treatment, I compiled information to ease the fears of future patients. My radiotherapy took just 28 seconds each day, which left me plenty of time to work on my project. I created a DVD with everything from taxi services to helpful local resources, which I distributed to doctor's offices and hospitals in Jersey. I felt like I had used my time well.

Many other patients, like me, were staying at the hotel, away from the comfort of home, and I knew many more would face the same situation in the future. Being far from home, often without family, is frightening. I wanted to ease some of that fear by gathering and organising as much helpful information as I could. If I could reduce the uncertainty for others, then every bit of research and support I provided felt worthwhile.

Chloë:

Not surprisingly, my mum had made friends in Southampton and settled in well. She'd even started writing notes and recording videos so the charity and the hospitals could share them with new cancer patients so they knew what to expect.

Mum's resilience was inspiring, and by the time she was declared cancer-free on my 21st birthday, it felt like a full-circle moment. It was the greatest gift I could have asked for.

Marilyn:

I had no effects from the radiotherapy other than a slight pink on my chest caused by it burning but it wasn't sore. I did not doubt in my mind that I would beat cancer and to have the all-clear on Chloë's special day, tells its own story.

Chloë:

I feel a strong sense of compassion for my younger self – a teenager on the brink of adulthood. Those were the years when I was beginning to explore my aspirations and ambitions, figuring out the kind of person I wanted to become.

It was vital to grant myself the space to simply be a young adult. I embraced the process of growing and evolving, allowing myself to heal through living life as normal as possible.

Marilyn:

The best advice I can give is to stay busy and keep your routine as normal as possible. Connect with others going through the same journey, as it helps to share experiences. Remember, cancer doesn't just affect you; it impacts your loved ones too. Be open about what you need from them.

My experience with cancer has made me appreciate life and realise how selfless so many people are. It has made me look at life differently and make every minute count. If you have a teen, make sure they know they are not alone and no matter what each day brings, you meet it with a smile.

Chloë:

If you're supporting someone with cancer, remember that listening is often the best thing you can do. Don't try to fix everything, just be there. At the same time, make sure you're looking after yourself too. You can't pour from an empty cup.

We're proud to share our story and hope it helps others in whatever way they need.

5

Letting Go to Move Forward

By Nicola George

Holy sh*t, I'm 40 and have breast cancer. Will I die?

Holy sh*t, I'm going through treatment during a pandemic. Will Covid kill me instead?

Holy sh*t, how am I supposed to stay positive for myself and my family?

Finding a lump at 40 was terrifying, but I tried to calm myself. Breast cancer doesn't happen to people who are young, fit and healthy, right? Well, wrong. I learned quickly that cancer doesn't care about any of that.

Sitting in that room with my husband, hearing the words, "You have breast cancer," is something that will stay with me forever. The first thing out of my mouth was, "Am I going to die?" Everything felt surreal. The words "treatable, chemotherapy, surgery" floated around, but nothing else made sense. Then I asked, "Will I lose my hair?" And the hardest question of all I didn't even dare speak: How do I explain this to my three daughters - aged

10, 17, and 20 – and my little boy, who's only 3, that mam has cancer and she's going to lose her hair?

I sat my kids down and did my best to keep it positive. But the moment I said "cancer," my 10-year-old, Ava, screamed. That word, to a child, means death. My older girls seemed okay at first, but as soon as the penny dropped that I'd lose my hair and get sick, the tears came.

My treatment plan was intense – eight months of chemotherapy, followed by a mastectomy and then radiotherapy. I had multiple lumps and two different types of cancer, so the chemo was split into two rounds: four sessions for one type and four for the other.

The first four sessions were of "The Red Devil" (that's what we call it). It's bright red, turns your wee red, and is so toxic it has to be injected by a nurse rather than a machine. One wrong move, and it could burn your skin off! The first couple of treatments were okay, but then the third session hit me like a ton of bricks. I had lost my hair, my skin was cracked and sore, and I looked like the stereotypical cancer patient.

Then came the second round, which we affectionately called "doce-tw*t-cel," a play on the name of the medication administered, docetaxel. Honestly, it was a tw*t. My joints ached, and it was like nothing I'd ever felt before. I felt like the Grand High Witch from Roald Dahl's *The Witches*, only without the disguise. By the time Session 8 rolled around, I'd had enough. My body gave up, and I did too. That's when I learned it's perfectly okay to say: "F*ck it". Sometimes, you have to prioritise yourself and let go of what feels impossible.

I was over the moon when my consultant agreed to skip the last step and go straight for the mastectomy. I opted for a full mastectomy with nipple removal; I wanted all of that trauma out of my life for good. No regrets. After surgery, I started a year of Herceptin injections every three weeks. And, hallelujah, I didn't need radiotherapy.

Throughout all this, my husband was my absolute rock. He took care of everything, never complaining, never showing his worry, except for one rare moment when he broke down. The kids understood what was happening and helped out, though my illness did take a toll. One of my daughters started self-harming, and another developed anorexia. It wasn't just cancer or Covid, but everything together didn't help.

Alongside my husband, my other guardian angel was Caroline, my breast care nurse. No question was too small, no worry too silly. She was always there, and I honestly don't know what I would've done without her.

The chemo ward became a second family, with patients and staff forming a little community. I never thought I'd say it, but when the treatments ended, I missed the people. Not the chemo, of course.

I vividly remember when Covid hit. I walked into the chemo ward, and the nurses, usually so full of smiles, were now hidden behind layers of PPE. Their eyes, usually kind, looked scared. It was unsettling when we had to move the chemo ward into a separate building – it felt terrifying. What kept me going through all of it was my twisted sense of humour and my blog Shitty Titties. Dark humour isn't for everyone, but it was my way of coping. It helped me, and apparently, it helped others too. People would tell me they felt braver going through their journeys because of my blog. That meant the world to me.

My kids shaved my head when the hair started falling out. I didn't like being "Nicola with cancer" every time I left the house, so I got a wig and felt more like myself again. The boost in confidence was unreal. On the rare occasions I felt well enough to go out, I'd end up swinging the wig around like a madwoman by the end of the night.

My Advice to Anyone Facing Cancer

Ask questions. Take a recorder to appointments if you have to. Use your breast care nurse - trust me, they are your lifeline. And read other people's stories, they'll help you feel less alone.

You get a card too when you join the Cancer Club. It's invisible but powerful. Housework? Can't, I have cancer. Food shop? Nope, cancer. Dinner? Sorry, I can't cook, cancer. No one can say no to you when you pull the cancer card! And the most important advice? Put things in the F*ck It Bucket. Let go of what doesn't matter. Cancer changes you - what once seemed important, now isn't.

People who drain you? Drop them. You get tougher. I even took some big risks during treatment, expanding my small childcare business into a private nursery with over a hundred children. Would I have had the guts to do that before? Nope.

Put yourself and your loved ones first, and focus on what truly matters. After all, we're warriors!

6

Calibrating Your Inner Radar:
Learning to Live with Uncertainty

By Dr. Peter Blackburn

Editor's note: Dr Blackburn is a Consultant Clinical Psychologist at the Bensham Hospital in Gateshead, UK. This is the metaphor he gives to his patients to help them understand and discern how to respond.

Think about the radar system used by air traffic control. The purpose of this radar is to monitor all planes in the airport's area. Air traffic control wants to know if all the planes are where they should be and that there are no dangers to its planes such as unregistered planes or hot air balloons etc. If air traffic control identifies one of these dangers, then it can sound the alarm.

Air traffic control needs to have radar with a helpful level of sensitivity, which identifies real dangers and is not too sensitive to identify a bird. If the radar is very sensitive and it identifies a bird as dangerous then it will be in a constant state of alarm and it will lead to the airport malfunctioning seeing everything as a danger.

Part of our brain known as the amygdala is designed to monitor and respond to threats in the outside world and our bodies. One of its roles is to ask: "Is it safe?"

When something frightening has happened to us, the amygdala's threat dial can be turned up because we can believe that we have been caught out by previous threats and we don't want to experience it again or we fear that the threat remains, and we are vulnerable in the future.

Therefore, we can get into a heightened state of anxiety through constantly monitoring and frequently identifying threats that are not dangerous. Constantly monitoring and living in a heightened state of alert can be exhausting and rob us of an enjoyable life. We go from living to fearfully existing, worrying that something bad is going to happen.

Part of the recovery process following a frightening experience is to courageously reset the sensitivity of our radar so that we can identify and respond to real dangers. Medical and nursing professionals can help you monitor for signs and symptoms that signify genuine danger. Any other signs and symptoms are likely to be normal sensations in your body - the equivalent of birds over the airport – which are identified by your radar as a threat when they are not.

The radar metaphor illustrates the normal monitoring we do and the anxiety we can feel but also how its sensitivity can be affected by frightening experiences and how it can then lead to us over-scanning our bodies looking for danger. The challenge is to reset it so that we identify genuine danger (based on discussions with nursing and medical professionals). This can be done by teaching yourself that there is no real danger, no tiger in the room, and learning to calm and soothe yourself, living fully, and learning to live with uncertainty.

Reflections from Nicola

Cancer can lead to denial, but accepting the reality of it is vital. Lauren's story shows that pushing for normality eventually becomes impossible, and emotional acknowledgement is key to healing.

Embracing physical changes after cancer, such as hair loss, can help regain control. Marie demonstrates how focusing on small victories, like styling wigs and small beauty routines, can restore confidence.

Caring for a loved one with cancer forces maturity. Laura's story emphasises resilience and the importance of stepping up during difficult times; while also acknowledging the emotional toll it takes on young carers.

Balancing self-care while supporting a loved one with cancer is crucial. Marilyn and Chloë highlight the need to maintain normal routines while also providing emotional support, and reminding others to take care of their mental health.

Sometimes it's necessary to let go and prioritise well-being over obligations. Nicola's humour and candidness about her struggles remind others that it's okay to drop what feels overwhelming and focus on healing. And don't forget your cancer card – the silver lining of Cancer Club.

Dr. Peter Blackburn's radar metaphor teaches us that past traumatic experiences can heighten our sensitivity to perceived threats, leading to constant vigilance. By resetting our "inner radar," we can learn to distinguish real dangers from false alarms, allowing us to live more fully and calmly amid uncertainty.

Chapter 2
Rediscovering the Self

There was a time during my treatment when I no longer felt like the extroverted, confident (sometimes over-confident) Nicola that I'd been my whole life. I had allowed cancer to crush me.

Seeing someone for the first time after they'd heard the news about my cancer was distressing for me. I hated the small talk. They felt as awkward as I did. The social complexities took so much out of me.

Simply going to Sainsbury's was like climbing Mount Everest. I would quickly get the shopping bags out of the car boot and then jump back inside and just sit. I would calm myself enough to get back out of the car and then feel the whoosh of panic and be unable to make it to the shop door. I would eventually make it into the shop but have to quickly turn around and leave without any shopping. I gave up even trying to venture to the supermarket and I didn't shop again for quite some time.

The gym was even scarier than Sainsbury's. Everybody knew me as "confident Nicola." Nicola who trains. Nicola who chats. Nicola who socialises. Nicola who spends loads of time talking in the changing rooms talking to everyone in just her knickers.

Although I was no stranger to fluctuation in my body weight over the years, the treatment began to impact me. My weight drastically changed, and so did my hormones. I sweated and panicked nonstop. I stopped going to the gym. I stopped going shopping. Slow, steady morning movement is crucial for preventing my rheumatoid arthritis flare-ups and I chose that pain over facing people at the gym, maintaining my fitness and the basic act of going food shopping.

I had let diagnosis become my identity. Everything felt like a sacrifice. It affected my fitness, my health, my career, my emotions, my life choices and my future.

When I heard the diagnosis, my life immediately revolved around cancer - hospital appointments, treatments, therapy, all on an endless loop. Cancer consumed me, eclipsing everything that made me who I was. The over-confident, extroverted Nicola faded into the background, and I let cancer take over. I wasn't just living with cancer; I was living cancer.

In the first few years following my cancer diagnosis, my arthritis was horrendous because I wasn't taking care of myself. Hormonal therapy took its toll and finally began to taper off; it was two years before I was able to feel ready to try and move again. The problem was that the old, confident Nicola had disappeared, and I knew I couldn't return to my original gym. I'd feel judged and pressured to be all bubbly and chatty like I used to be. I didn't want them to know the truth, that on the inside I was a wreck, crying myself to sleep at night, crippled with anxiety about what was happening. I decided to find a new gym.

Steve took me to visit all the local gyms until I found one - a posh one with retired folk where I wouldn't have to stay and chat, where no one knew me and nobody would ask me questions or stare at me. Cancer Club paranoia, another delightful side benefit.

My siblings and friends had gotten used to doing the shopping for me, bless them. We took it slowly and started with baby steps; Steve would drive me to a shop in another part of town. At first, I would stay in the car while he did the shopping. Gradually, I built up the confidence to go in by myself. I was so terrified of bumping into someone I knew and seeing how they would look at me with pity as they asked me probing questions about my health. I didn't want anyone to say something inappropriate in front of my little boy, so I created what felt like a secret plan with Steve to visit different shops away from where we lived.

My inner circle was small – my husband, son, brother, sister, a few close friends and family. I started to realise I was isolating myself like Harry Potter locked away in the cupboard. I missed being outside. Steve would encourage me to go for a drive, far enough from home so I wouldn't run into anyone and have to deal with awkward, stressful conversations. Fresh air has always been a great pick-me-up, and once we arrived somewhere far enough away, I could relax, breathe deeply, and let it cleanse my lungs. It felt like a brief escape, as if I'd been let out of jail and I savoured that short freedom before heading back to reality.

Living near the coast has always been good for my soul. The beach is my happy place. My best memories are at the beach. When I was avoiding people, Steve or a friend would drive me there super early. Sitting on an empty beach in the early hours, listening to the waves crash and feeling the wind on my face, grounded me. It would take me back to being a little girl. It allowed me to drift away into those special, happy times and escape for a while.

In my opinion, nothing makes you feel better than a cuddle. I heard somewhere that if you cuddle somebody for 20 seconds, magic happens. I used to practise 20-second cuddles with my son, Gabriel. Your breathing starts to align, you feel relaxed and your troubles begin to melt away. Nothing calms me down more than a 20-second cuddle.

Slowly, I started to regain pieces of myself. Little rituals like colouring became moments of calm. With every stroke of colour, I could focus on something beyond my diagnosis. Everything slowed down – my racing thoughts, my "what ifs" – and for a little while, it was just me, the colours, and the paper. It was in these small acts, whether it was a long hug with my son or scribbling in a colouring book, that I started to reclaim control over my life.

Another way that helped me cope was through planning. I love planning. There was so much uncertainty around treatments and appointments – I would find ways to control things by organising my schedule. My notebook was always close to hand so I could make a note of any questions that I wanted to ask at the hospital. My little lists helped me feel prepared for my hospital appointments. They gave me comfort. Looking back, I realise it was a way of controlling what I could. Every small bit of control you can hold onto makes you feel better.

I began writing and discovered a new-found love for it. I don't write to win prizes – I write because it is therapeutic for me. In the evenings, I could not switch myself off from the "what ifs." I would have a tiny thought that would grow arms and legs and become the biggest, scariest scenario ever. Every question that popped in, I would write down. Spending time reflecting on these started to show me how crazy they were.

Writing things down at bedtime, rather than letting them grow in my mind, helped me get to sleep. I started using this process in the mornings too, journalling my feelings. I wondered if there was a book out there that could answer all of my questions – there wasn't and there never will be. Here I am creating this book for you to read.

Inviting you into the crevices of my mind, the collective experiences of the stories that unfold on the pages. It won't answer all of your questions, but it may go some way to knowing that you are not alone.

As I started to rebuild myself, I discovered the world of self-development (thanks to Angela Walton, Paul Mort, the Inner Circle ladies, and my daily accountability heroes). I now know what things work for me: exercise, fresh air, meditation, eating well, talking, journalling, writing, and taking days off. Before cancer, I didn't do any of this. I pushed myself at a million miles an hour until I eventually collapsed, unable to maintain that pace.

In the end, finding peace wasn't about conquering the unknown, it was about savouring those moments when the wind hit my face at the beach, or when my son and I shared those magical 20-second hugs that made the world feel just a little less heavy.

What follows are stories about failure, trial, failure again, and success. These are tales on how to avoid perpetual victimhood, over-planning, over-thinking, and over-anything. It's about living with uncertainty.

7

Letting Go of Control to Embrace the Present

By Carmel Watson

Most days, I live in a world full of sunshine and positivity. But there are times when I walk under a dark storm cloud that threatens to drench me. No matter how much I try to outrun it, the rain cloud keeps pace, following my every step. That's what living with terminal cancer feels like.

In spring 2020, after months of pain in my back and knee, I finally broke down at work. I had been back and forth to the doctor with little relief. This time, a nurse decided to send my blood off for testing, just to be sure. Two days later, I got a call. Three raised indicators which were signs of inflammation. Further tests revealed a mass growing near my spine.

I remember the date vividly – 16 April 2020, my 63rd birthday – when I had an endoscopy. Not exactly the birthday present I had imagined. Soon after, I sat with my daughter in a room with Mr. French, a surgeon at Freeman Hospital. He explained, quite plainly, that a rare and slow-growing sarcoma was attacking my body. I wasn't entirely prepared for the list of organs they'd have to remove. My left kidney, my gallbladder, my spleen, even parts of my pancreas – each one more shocking than the last.

The surgery was eight and a half hours. The surgeon told me not to be alarmed when I came around as I would have more tubes coming out of me than the back of a television set – he didn't exaggerate. After a few days, I was moved out of the ICU and into a main ward. But even through those dark days in the hospital, I found moments of humour.

One night, I accidentally triggered a medical alarm with my toiletries bag, sending a dozen frantic medics into the room. "Sorry about that," I muttered, while they all shuffled away, complaining that they had just been about to take a bite of their sandwich. I didn't think much of it, but the other women in the ward were in absolute hysterics at my nonchalant attitude. It's not that I wasn't sorry for causing the panic – I just hadn't done it on purpose. I didn't mean to cause chaos, but we had a good laugh.

In the ward, I met some other lovely patients and the most wonderful, kind, and caring nursing staff, who truly were angels. I remember one nurse took me into the shower, sat me on a plastic chair, and washed my hair for me late one night because I had been unable to do it myself due to feeling dizzy. She was just one of a host of staff who went over and beyond the call of duty.

Upon my discharge from the Freeman Hospital, I was told by the surgeon that he was happy they had successfully removed all the tumour and that there would be no need for any chemo or radiotherapy. Regular CT scans were to follow to ensure no recurrence.

Fast forward three years. All my scans had been clear until May 2023. That's when I got the news - another tumour, this time inoperable, growing on what was left of my pancreas. When my surgeon told me that my life expectancy might not be measured in years, but in months, it felt like a punch to the stomach. I was stunned, but I wasn't ready to give up.

In August, I started palliative chemotherapy with Dr. Beth, who has a soothing voice and gives me hope. We hoped the chemo would shrink the tumour, but it didn't. During the chemotherapy, I was expecting nausea, hair loss, and fatigue. I also developed painful mouth ulcers. I was prescribed various mouthwashes, sprays, and gels but nothing worked until I discovered aloe vera gel, which thankfully eased the symptoms. By Christmas, we decided to stop treatment temporarily to give my body a break. Dr. Beth looked me in the eye and said, "You're strong in your head, but your body is frail." That stuck with me.

In January 2024, I was admitted to have a port fitted for intravenous administration of chemotherapy, and blood taken through one tube. Since the port was completely hidden under my skin it was less likely to become infected. Trabectedin was administered, not to reduce the size of the tumour but to hopefully stop it from growing too big too quickly. As I write this, I am done with two treatments – the tumour continues to grow but I am hopeful that after further treatments this may improve.

Despite all this, I don't feel ill. Most people wouldn't even know I have cancer if I didn't tell them. I still enjoy regular walks and a cuppa or two with my friends and family, and my grandchildren light up my days.

I even go to the local hospice, St. Benedict's in Ryhope, once a week as part of a 12-week session. I've been absolutely loving it as the staff are fabulous, and I have made new friends along the way. Life goes on.

I've stopped worrying about the things I can't control. Instead, I wake up each morning, thank God for another day, and try to live fully in the present. I don't know how much time I have left, but I do know this: I'm going to spend it surrounded by the people I love.

Life is good.

8

Operating on Autopilot:
A Survival Mechanism

By Sophie Ryan

Each year on the anniversary of Mum's passing, I write her a letter. It's my way of updating her on all that's happened. As I type, the tears flow freely, every emotion pouring out - grief, love, memories. It's my release, a chance to say everything I wish I could tell her in person.

Mum, who we affectionately called The Mothership, started feeling pain in her sides and became short of breath. A scan revealed what we all feared: a shadow on her lungs. She was a lifelong smoker, so deep down, we knew what it meant. My twin sister and dad were overwhelmed with emotion, while my brother, who had been on holiday, returned to the devastating news. Day by day, we all rallied around Mum, visiting her and Dad regularly, though my sister handled most of the daily caregiving. As for me, I slipped into autopilot, managing the situation the only way I knew how by staying focused and getting through each day.

We didn't realise at the time that we only had five months left with her. Mum wasn't a fighter by nature, and chemo was incredibly hard on her. She stopped eating and lost so much weight. It wasn't just her body that suffered, her mental state faded too, and it was heartbreaking to watch her withdraw from us, especially from her grandkids, with whom she had been so close. Watching that bond fade was one of the hardest things.

Her hair began to thin and fall out, but wigs didn't matter to my mum. She wasn't fussed about appearances; she only bought a couple of head towels. The chemo reduced the cancer by 80%, but it also triggered paraneoplastic syndrome, which affected her brain. The woman who had always been so present was slipping away before our eyes.

One day, I was rushing to pick up my kids from school when I got the call. "Come now," they said. I didn't think it would be so sudden, so I didn't rush. By the time I arrived, I was 15 minutes too late. Mum was already gone. I wrapped her up in blankets, instinctively trying to keep her warm. The finality of it was surreal.

Everyone handles cancer differently. My sister and dad wore their emotions openly, but I stayed practical.

That's how I coped, focusing on what needed to be done. Mum and I even planned her funeral together in her final days, which was oddly comforting. It felt right that she had a say in how she would be remembered, and it gave me something concrete to focus on.

In the days following her death, I felt anger creeping in. While others cried, I found myself thinking, "I need to call Mum - it's been a while." Then the reality would hit hard: I couldn't call her. The real grief struck during the children's first birthdays without her. The fact that she would never again witness those precious moments, that's when the loss felt the deepest.

Supporting someone with cancer teaches you to value the body, fragile as it is. We all know it's not forever, but witnessing it firsthand brings that truth painfully close. I stayed on autopilot through most of her illness, but writing her these letters each year has been my way of reconnecting with my emotions, of grieving in my own time. They sit quietly on my computer, like a diary of our family's life since Mum left.

There's no "right" way to handle something as massive as cancer. It comes with a whirlwind of emotions - fear, anger, sadness, and yes, sometimes numbness.

If autopilot helps get you through, then that's okay. But finding space to let those emotions out, in whatever form that takes, is just as important.

9

"Why Not Me?": Facing Cancer Without Victimhood

By Celia Samater

I was living what I thought was the perfect life in Saudi Arabia - dream job, happy family, everything in its place. So when I got my cancer diagnosis, my first thought was how *inconvenient* it all was! Death didn't cross my mind; I was more focused on fitting treatment into my already busy life. Meanwhile, my husband had the opposite reaction; he was already planning my funeral and thinking about how it would affect our boys, aged 12 and 8.

In Saudi, I had a great oncologist, but finding the right surgeon was a nightmare. I spent months in and out of tests and consultations. Eventually, I returned to the UK for a lumpectomy, intending to finish treatment back in Saudi. But that wasn't to be. During my first UK appointment, they discovered the whole right breast was affected. I would need a full mastectomy. That was a shock. But true to my nature, I didn't panic - I simply recalculated how to manage everything.

After the surgery, I went back to Saudi and continued working while trying to coordinate the next steps. My husband and I faced the impossible choice of staying there for treatment or coming home to the UK without him. I chose to return to the UK with our boys. In a matter of weeks, everything changed – my dream life had blown apart. Thankfully, I had a strong support network in the UK, but it wasn't easy.

Treatment was anything but smooth. I went through the full works: chemo, radiotherapy, and multiple surgeries. I lost my hair, battled sickness and became a paranoid insomniac for five days every three weeks. But you just keep going; there's no other choice.

The boys took everything in their stride, and having them at home with me helped create a routine and purpose. Work was kind enough to let me continue remotely when I could manage it. My husband stayed in Saudi, but the separation was one of the hardest things for us to deal with.

I never wasted energy asking, "Why me?" It's a pointless question. I focused on what was in front of me because if I kept going, so would the boys. My mindset was all about shielding them from unnecessary worry. Even with them at home, it was still heartbreaking to be separated from our family unit.

After chemo, I insisted on an immediate reconstruction. My surgeon advised against it, but I wanted it done. Well, it turned out the surgeon was right - four days later, I was in A&E with nerve damage and cellulitis. My body rejected the implant, and after multiple surgeries, I ended up with no implant and no right breast. But at that point, I had no energy left to mourn that loss. I was just grateful to get through the summer, practically living in Queen Elizabeth Hospital.

Six years on, I've had more surgeries, and I'm five years into Tamoxifen. Although I finally have two breasts, they're mismatched, and my body's a patchwork of scars. But hey, I did get a tummy tuck and some bonus liposuction in the process - silver linings, right?

I couldn't have made it through without my husband. I still remember the day he surprised me by flying in from Saudi for a chemo session, the nurses were crying like it was a scene from a movie. My support system also included my mother, mother-in-law, and my closest friends. Julie, especially, always had me in stitches with her dark humour. Anytime we went out, she'd whisper,

"Have you got your cancer card for a discount?" It was laughter like that which kept me sane.

Of course, not everyone knew how to handle the news. One friend avoided me for two weeks because she didn't know what to say. When I finally saw her, I made a joke about how contagious I was. That broke the ice. Humour and honesty became my greatest tools for navigating awkwardness.

The turning point came when I got my first real-hair wig from The Wonderful Wig Company. Nicola Wood, the founder, took me under her wing, and it was a game-changer. I looked like myself again, which did wonders for my confidence. It's amazing how important it is to be able to feel like my old self – not "the cancer patient."

Mindset Is Everything

Throughout this journey, I never asked, "Why me?" I made a pact with myself: Asking that question was the same as wishing this on someone else and I couldn't do that. I believed I could get through it, and I was right.

Gratitude became my lifeline. On days when I felt sorry for myself, I would read notes of encouragement and look at the gifts I'd been given. They reminded me that even in the darkest times, there are always reasons to be grateful.

Running and eating healthy were my ways of taking control. While the medical team did their job, this was how I could do mine. Slowly, I rebuilt not just my body, but my sense of purpose. I studied coaching, earned my NLP Life Coaching qualification, and started working on my website, determined to use my experience to help others.

Today, I have my family, my health, and my career. What more could I ask for? The key to getting through cancer – or anything really – is mindset. Be positive. Be thankful. And never, ever stop moving forward.

10

The Power of Community in the Face of Illness

By Donna Stewart

Editor's note: Donna Stewart sadly passed away on 22 June 2024. Below are her own words about her journey followed by a note from her daughter, Georgia Sutton.

I had been suffering from unbearable headaches for days when a friend took me to A&E. My GP thought it was just a migraine, but a scan revealed a brain tumour the size of a small orange. That same night, I was in surgery. They managed to remove 80% of the tumour, but due to its location, the rest was too risky to take out.

The reality sank in over the following days – where there's a tumour, there's often cancer. When I was diagnosed with an aggressive form, the shock rippled through my family and friends. But I didn't let myself get upset; I just kept moving forward, determined to face treatment head-on.

Radiotherapy came first: 28 sessions of being bolted into a head mask and strapped down on a table. It was unsettling but necessary. After that, I faced six months of chemotherapy. Chemo made me violently sick, and the steroids caused me to put on about four stone. On top of everything, losing my independence was a huge blow. I had to surrender my driving licence and rely on others for transport, which was hard to adjust to. But I was surrounded by people who stepped in to help.

Throughout this journey, my loved ones always coped and supported me. My husband, understandably, couldn't shake off the negativity wholly, but I tried to stay positive for both of us.

Despite the challenges, I found ways to cope. Spending time with friends, and going on holidays when I could. It was those moments of normality that kept me feeling like myself. One of the most empowering experiences was participating in Courage on the Catwalk, a fashion show for cancer patients. Strutting down that runway made me feel strong and less alone, surrounded by people who knew what I was going through.

How the Rest of the Story Unfolded

Humour became my lifeline. After my diagnosis, I treated myself to a Dyson Air Wrap, a little indulgence. Then I realised I wouldn't have any hair to style and burst out laughing! I joked with my husband too, teasing him, "Your new wife won't be getting my new ironing board!" I could sense that my husband was dealing with his feelings of isolation as a supporter, so I made a conscious effort to reassure him that despite the challenges, I was still the same person and that we were in this together.

Even though cancer has impacted my career, forcing me to stop working since 2019, I still managed to tick off one of my dreams. Last year, I completed a tandem skydive, raising over £19,000 for charity with a group of amazing people. I also bought a static home in Spain, where I've been able to spend precious time with family and friends. And I'm looking forward to a cruise around the Arctic later this year.

Through it all, my family and friends have been my greatest support. Nicola, who rushed me to A&E that first day, Sandra, who took me to every radiotherapy appointment, and my brother, who handled all the legal matters – I owe so much to them. And my children, my heart and soul, have kept me focused on what's most important: family. When my daughter told me she was pregnant not long after my diagnosis, I feared I wouldn't meet my grandchild. Now, he's three, and I've been blessed with another grandson, too. They bring me such happiness.

Staying Positive and Connected

Positivity and connection are everything when facing cancer. Loneliness can be one of the hardest parts of this journey, but reaching out to others who understand can make all the difference. Online communities, Facebook groups, and forums are incredible resources – they help you feel less alone and more empowered to face each day.

Ask as many questions as you need to. Medical jargon can be overwhelming, and it's important to understand what's happening with your body. And remember, when it comes to your prognosis, you are not just a statistic.

Always have something to look forward to. It doesn't have to be a big event like a trip to the moon or a date with Brad Pitt. Sometimes a simple coffee with friends can make all the difference. And remember, don't pay attention to the people who suddenly think they're trained oncologists!

A note from Donna's daughter, Georgia:

We lost mum on 22 June 2024. I only found out that she had contributed to this book after stumbling upon an email from Nicola with the subject line, "Cancer book update." I was confused but excited, so I called Nicola and asked what it was all about. I had no idea Mum had written anything for this book, but getting to read her unfiltered story now that she is gone feels like such a gift.

"Since you passed, Mum, it's been hard to adjust to life without your smile or your comforting laugh. So many of us still find it hard to believe you're not here. I hope we've made you proud in the time since you left us. I think about you every day and how brave you were throughout your cancer journey. I know you must have had moments of sadness and worry that you didn't share with us, but you always put on the bravest face. You were the strongest woman I have ever known, and I'm so proud to call you, my mum. My heart breaks knowing you'll miss out on so much, especially when it comes to your grandchildren, but I promise we will keep your memory alive. We love and miss you so much, Mum – you truly were one of a kind."

11

Strength in Guilt and Grace

By Andy Nisevic

Despite my nan's breast cancer being diagnosed in the early stages, the emotional toll was immense. The necessity of a mastectomy weighed heavily on her psyche. For a woman who had always been so sure of herself, it was a hard pill to swallow. But my nan, a strong-willed Eastern European woman, decided to go ahead with the surgery. It wasn't easy, but she believed it was the right choice. The surgery was a success, and, remarkably, no further treatment was necessary. We all breathed a sigh of relief.

But just as we began to embrace the news of Nan's recovery, my grandad received his diagnosis: life-limiting pancreatic cancer. By the time they found it, the cancer had already infiltrated his lymph nodes. It was advanced, and there was nothing they could do.

My nan had always been the strong matriarch of the family. In our Eastern European Orthodox culture, the role of the matriarch is to nurture and support everyone else. It's a heavy burden to carry. Even though Nan had just come through her own battle with cancer, she now had to watch her husband face his. She confided in me through tear-filled eyes, the first time I'd ever seen her cry and explain that she felt guilty. Guilt that she had chosen surgery for herself, that she had survived. She said that if she had known what was coming for my grandad, she would have made a different decision. She would have faced cancer alongside him and foregone her surgery so they could go through it together. It broke my heart to see her struggle with that.

My nan threw herself into the role of caregiver for my grandad. It wasn't easy. She didn't drive, so she relied on family members to take her and grandad to medical appointments and run errands. Despite this, she never complained. She simply did what she had to do. That was her way, just getting on with things, no matter how hard it was. My dad stepped in to help in the "man's role," as grandad could no longer handle any physical tasks around the house. But the emotional and mental toll fell on my nan.

One of the few people Nan seemed comfortable leaning on during this time was my dad's ex-wife. Though no longer married to my dad, she and Nan had developed a deep bond over the years. Their shared experiences as women navigating marriages with, shall we say, "old-fashioned" mentalities, had brought them closer. My dad's ex-wife became a pillar of emotional support for Nan during Grandad's illness. It's funny how those relationships we might not expect can end up being the most valuable.

The Struggle with Guilt and Sacrifice

Looking back now, I see my nan's approach as both admirable and concerning. On one hand, she was a testament to strength, showing all of us what it means to push forward despite the weight of the world on our shoulders. On the other hand, I can't help but wonder if she was truly happy. She embodied the old-fashioned notion of silently enduring hardship. That's what kept her going, but I think it also meant she put everyone else's needs above her own. In the end, it cost her.

As I've grown older, I've come to realise how deeply survival guilt affected her. She overextended herself, always giving and caring for others while neglecting her well-being. It was as if she believed that by surviving cancer, she owed it to the world to care for my grandad and keep the family together, no matter the toll it took on her emotionally and mentally. I wish I had known more about mental health and mindset back then. I would have encouraged her to seek support, to connect with others who had gone through similar experiences. Maybe that would have helped her process the guilt and find some peace.

Though I was young at the time, this period in our family's life stands out to me. It taught me two powerful lessons. First, human beings are capable of extraordinary things when we apply ourselves, especially in the face of hardship. My nan's resilience showed me that. Second, the sacrifices we make, especially when we do them silently, can have long-term impacts that we may not fully understand until much later.

It is a reminder that life is short, and guilt doesn't help anyone. My nan's guilt, though understandable, only made her journey harder. If there's one thing I've learned, it's that you deserve joy, too. You deserve to find what makes you happy and pursue it without guilt. You are more capable and deserving of happiness than you may realise. My nan taught me that strength doesn't just come from enduring; it comes from knowing when to take care of yourself as well.

12

Fighting for Myself and My Children

By Sarah Helaine Moniz

This year, I'm celebrating both my 50th and my 5th "birthday" of survival. It feels surreal to be here, alive and thriving. Surviving cancer gave me the motivation to truly live my best life. I've moved to a new home, opened two businesses, and even fulfilled my dream of becoming a medium.

My story, however, doesn't begin with my diagnosis. It begins with my former husband Andrew. He was diagnosed with pancreatic cancer after a trip to A&E. We had no idea what was coming. He had just undergone a series of tests a week earlier, but somehow, his results had been missed. By the time the cancer was discovered, it had already spread to his liver, bowel, and spine.

Coming from a medical family, I knew the seriousness of this diagnosis. I remember sitting on the children's climbing frame in the garden, trying to shield our kids from the conversation, as Andrew told me the devastating news. His initial reaction was denial, but I had already braced myself for what was coming.

Andrew's treatment had been palliative for pancreatic cancer. His condition degenerated quickly. Within days, Andrew requested to be moved to a hospice, Priscilla Bacon Lodge in Norwich. I gave up my job so I could take the children to visit him after school. They found it difficult, and my younger son didn't want to eat. Not wanting people to see him suffer, Andrew declined visitors other than his children. Andrew passed away peacefully in the evening, five weeks after his diagnosis.

Navigating My Diagnosis

Just over a year after Andrew passed, and two weeks after our children had finished bereavement counselling, I found a lump in my breast. It was surreal. The timing couldn't have been worse. We had barely begun adjusting to life without Andrew when I got my cancer diagnosis. My maternal instinct kicked in. I knew I was all my children had left, and I was determined not to give up. My fight became about them, not just me.

When my eldest daughter asked if I had cancer and was going to die too, I reassured her. Dad's cancer had been found too late, but mine had been caught before it could spread. I promised my kids that I would never stop fighting, and I meant it.

Balancing Treatment and Motherhood

The lead-up to Christmas after my diagnosis felt unreal. Everything around me seemed distant. While everyone was caught up in holiday excitement, I was wondering if this would be my last Christmas. My treatment was intense. I underwent a mastectomy, and later, 6 rounds of chemotherapy and 15 radiotherapy sessions. But I had a team of incredible supporters: my kids, my parents, my friends. They built me a four-poster bed, stocked my fridge, and kept my home running while I focused on healing.

After my mastectomy, I had a Velcro wrap around my chest and a drain bag that my friend cleverly hid in a pretty biscuit tin to make it easier to carry around. The younger kids and the cat went to a friend's house so I could rest, and my friend stayed the first night on the sofa. The next day, after she left, I tottered into the kitchen, tin in hand, crying but determined to make a cup of tea, a small but powerful moment where I fought to stay strong. Another friend had kindly stocked my fridge with ready meals.

Balancing my health with the emotional needs of my children was the hardest part. I had to be there for them even when I could barely stand. Some days, I didn't think I had it in me, but the unwavering support of my family and friends kept me going. My father drove me to my first chemo session, which just happened to fall on my 45th birthday. I wasn't thrilled about the needles, but I made it through with my crystal angel in hand and my dad by my side. I managed to cope whilst my dad chatted over the crossword.

My main challenge was coping with the effects of the drugs, which were doing their job of eradicating any remaining cells that had escaped the mastectomy. For about five days after each treatment, I felt pretty rough.

My days revolved around seeing my children off to high school and enjoying visits from wonderful friends. Walking any distance was difficult, and I only went out during the recovery weeks of the chemotherapy cycle.

By the time I reached the radiotherapy sessions, I was driving again. After my final appointment with the consultant in August, I rang the bell.

Creating a New Normal

Post-treatment life wasn't easy, but I was determined to recover in style. I set up my recovery space downstairs, transformed our dining room into my bedroom and even hired a cleaner. Slowly but surely, I regained my strength.

The hardest part wasn't the treatment itself, it was adjusting to the changes in my body. Losing my hair and dealing with medical menopause and nerve damage took time to accept.

My old self didn't return when my hair grew back. The red hair I had before cancer never returned, but I've learned to embrace the new me. My once wispy, thin hair is now dyed purple – because why not? It's a symbol of the new version of myself I've grown to love.

What Helped Me Along the Way

Through it all, I learned some valuable lessons. Understanding that cancer isn't your fault helps. Knowing that anyone can fall victim to rogue cells makes it a little less personal.

I found comfort in small things, like using binaural beats to ease my nausea and indulging in a big breakfast when that's what my body craved. I even had a glass of red wine on the nights before my chemo.

Most importantly, I learned to make space for joy. My kids loved snuggling up to watch TV in my recovery room, and I cherished those moments.

I rewarded myself after each chemo session, whether with a small gift or a special meal. And I made sure my recovery space felt pampering, filled with warmth and love.

At my local hospital, a cancer charity help centre provided a quiet space for me to rest between treatments, offering plenty of cuppas and a sympathetic ear. They also arranged complimentary treatments from a reflexologist and a Reiki master. My hobby of tribal belly dancing helped me regain movement after surgery, as I practised arm movements to prevent cording.

My spiritual community and personal practices were a strong source of support. As a Reiki Master, Crystal Healer, and Medium, I was already in training before my diagnosis. Meditation became a key part of my routine, helping to distract me from discomfort and improve my sleep.

Gifts made me feel special. One was a set of beautiful costume jewellery and clothes from a neighbour of my mum's. I felt pretty despite the bald head. The second was a box from Little Lifts that contained lots of little helpful things such as plain lotions and bamboo toothbrushes that helped me to cope with the daily challenges of treatment effects.

If there's one piece of advice I'd give to anyone going through this, it's to take each day as it comes. Don't shy away from asking for help. Your strength is not just in fighting the disease but in allowing others to help you along the way.

Living in the Present

I'm now five years in remission, but I know this journey has shaped me in ways that go beyond the physical scars. Watching my children grow and thrive, despite the trauma of losing their father and nearly losing me, has given me a deep sense of gratitude. The closeness we've built as a family is a gift I'll always treasure.

A cancer diagnosis is not necessarily a death sentence anymore. Breast cancer can be spotted and treated quickly. Modern cancer treatments can and do help overcome this disease. My advice is please get checked. It is better to be wrong than too late.

There's something profoundly ironic yet beautiful about facing your mortality, it teaches you to live fully in the present. And for that, I am grateful.

13

Living in the Now,
Not in Fear of Tomorrow

By Gabrielle Mottershead

When my treatment ended, I expected to feel relief, maybe even triumph. Instead, I fell apart. I was exhausted, weepy, and terrified of recurrence. I had beaten cancer, but now I faced a new battle, learning how to live without constant fear.

My diagnosis in 2008 was a shock. I didn't have a lump, just a thickening of the skin, and yet, that small change turned out to be inflammatory breast cancer - rare, aggressive, and life-altering. I was 44, healthy, and suddenly thrown into a whirlwind of high-dose chemotherapy, a mastectomy, and radiotherapy. Everything happened so fast; it was like I was on autopilot, just trying to get through it all. Eighteen months later, I underwent a breast reconstruction, where a piece of my stomach was used to create a new breast.

Paul, my husband, was amazing. He came to every appointment, shaved my head when the hair started falling out, and told me I was beautiful even when I felt like I looked like a bloated alien from all the steroids. We spent long days in bed, watching *Desperate Housewives* and pretending that life was still normal, even though it was far from it.

Losing my hair during chemo was devastating. I remember going into Boots for a sandwich and wearing a headscarf because I was completely bald. When I paid, they handed me a receipt and a voucher for money off shampoo. I was livid! I can't recall what I said, but I was so angry and upset that the poor sales assistant was speechless. I still feel bad for my outbursts and tears.

The Weight of Beating Cancer

But when it was all over, I wasn't prepared for how lost I would feel. The anxiety was paralysing. Every ache and every pain made me think the cancer was back. I couldn't sleep, constantly terrified of what might be hiding inside my body. Adding to my distress was the realisation that my career, which I had sacrificed so much for, suddenly felt meaningless. I had poured years into my job, driven by relentless stress and pressure. Reflecting on it now, I see how that toxic work environment had been chipping away at my health long before the cancer came.

Sixteen years later, I know now that what I was experiencing wasn't just fear - it was PTSD. The trauma of cancer, the endless treatments and the mental strain had left deep scars. But once I recognised that, I was able to start healing.

Confidence After Cancer

The turning point came when I realised that, after everything I had been through, I needed to take care of *myself* first. That's not something many women are taught to do, especially if they're used to being caregivers. Louise Hay's book *You Can Heal Your Life* was a game changer for me. It taught me that you can't pour from an empty cup; self-love and self-care are essential.

I threw myself into recovery, studying everything from nutritional healing to Reiki, breathwork, and coaching. I realised my biggest battle wasn't against cancer anymore, it was against fear. Slowly but surely, I rebuilt my confidence and learned how to live without that constant anxiety looming over me.

Many of the people I support now through Confidence After Cancer tell me they feel the same. They've beaten the disease, but they're stuck in fear, unable to imagine a future. I know that feeling well, and that's why I founded this community. Through our website, podcast and social platforms, we share what it takes to live well after treatment ends.

We focus on healing not just the body, but the mind and soul, too.

Today, I'm happy, healthy, and doing what I love, helping others navigate their post-cancer journeys. If you're reading this and your treatment has ended but you feel like no one understands, know that I'm here for you. Recovery is about so much more than just surviving. It's about learning to live fully again, without fear holding you back.

Reflections from Nicola

Carmel's journey demonstrates the power of letting go of what cannot be controlled and focusing on what truly matters. The more life-limiting the condition is, the more clarity and peace people seem to have. It comes with a level of acceptance that Carmel demonstrates beautifully.

Operating on autopilot can help survive the immediacy of grief, but finding moments to release emotions is key for long-term healing as Sophie showed.

Refusing to adopt a victim mentality, Celia explains, and focusing on practical solutions can provide strength for both oneself and one's family during cancer treatment.

Donna's experience highlights the power of community and surrounding yourself with people who love and support you, easing the loneliness and fear that cancer brings.

Survivor's guilt can be an unseen emotional burden but resilience is found in self-sacrifice, cultural expectations, and ultimately the grace to prioritise others while confronting challenges.

Sarah's unrelenting determination to survive for her children reveals the overwhelming power of love and responsibility in conquering life's darkest moments.

Gabrielle teaches us that living fully in the moment, rather than dwelling on the fear of cancer returning, brings more joy and freedom than ever before.

Collectively, these stories remind us that cancer is not just a physical fight. It's emotional, psychological, and deeply personal, requiring strength, community, and the courage to embrace life, no matter what challenges come your way.

Chapter 3
Looking in the Mirror

I screamed an unrepeatable name at Steve as I slammed the car door. My poor husband just sat there looking bewildered. Five weeks of daily radiotherapy had worn me down - mind, body and spirit. The weight of it all was crushing. I had been crying from the moment I woke up that day and throughout the car ride to the hospital. Maybe it was because Gabriel wasn't with us that day, so I didn't need to put on a brave face. I just didn't want to go. I hated that I *had* to go. Everything felt sh*t and Steve was the closest person that I could lash out on.

To his credit, he was an absolute angel - but something snapped in me that day. I called him a terrible name. I had never called him anything like that before and never have since, but just that one time, I played my cancer card and got away with it.

As if that wasn't enough, I forbid him from coming into the hospital with me. "You're not coming in. I'm doing it on my own," I yelled at him. Of course, I didn't want to do it alone. I wanted him by my side, but in my anger, I wanted him to hurt because I was hurting. I knew that later I could twist it, accuse him of not caring enough, simply because he respected my request. What a b*tch, eh?

I stormed across the hospital car park and marched into the radiotherapy department in full meltdown mode. I lay on the bed, sobbing, my body shaking while the radiographers lined up the lasers to hit my tattooed dots. I couldn't move, but inside, I was spiralling. And those small black dots - symbols of this club membership that I never asked for - felt like a reminder that nothing would ever be the same again. Little did I know how symbolic these small black dots would become.

When I finally emerged, there was Steve, tentatively waiting for me, as I knew he would be. He didn't listen when I told him to stay away, because he knew better. As soon as I saw him, I collapsed into his arms, crying again. He held me tight, and I let myself fall apart.

As you've probably guessed by now, I'm an intense sort of person. Steve knows me better than anyone. He's been there for every breakdown, and somehow, he always knows what I need. There were many moments like this throughout my journey, and through it all, he stayed, as did my family and close friends. I was lucky. They made me feel loved, even as cancer stripped so much away from me.

But no matter how much love I felt from them, loving *myself* became the hardest part. I looked in the mirror, and the reflection staring back wasn't the Nicola I knew. Cancer had changed me, and not just in the obvious ways. I wasn't one of those people who handled treatment by hitting the gym and eating healthily. Self-care went out the window. I was the person who ate packet after packet of Hobnobs, justifying it with, "I have cancer; I'll eat what I want!" Week by week, my body grew softer and rounder. My face filled out, and I felt less like *me* with every day that passed.

For someone who had spent her life working in the hairdressing industry, hair was everything! Even though I didn't lose my hair, the fear of "What if?" hovered over me constantly. Hair was my career - my life. I had spent years making people feel beautiful with their hair. How could I be "Nic the hairdresser" if I didn't have my own? That thought was almost more terrifying than the cancer itself.

To set the record straight, I was fortunate I did not lose my hair - this is the most dreaded side effect of chemo. The most common preconception people have about why I set up my business is around my hair loss. I'm asked during podcasts, interviews, and award ceremonies: "Did you lose your hair?" My answer is simple: "No, I didn't." But that didn't take away the fear of "What if?" My entire life was hair, every day surrounded by mirrors and hair - both mine and my clients. How could I be Nicola if I did not have my hair?

Although chemotherapy wasn't required in the end, it was never guaranteed at the start. With invasive cancer, I had to wait until after my lumpectomy, when they examined the area and removed my sentinel lymph nodes, to see if it had spread. Until then, everything hung in the balance. I'm deeply grateful, but the relief only came after a long period of uncertainty - nothing was promised from the beginning.

Over the years, changes in my arthritis medication meant I had to take some pretty harsh drugs. These medications caused my hair in my twenties and thirties to become dry, brittle and shed significantly. I had quietly struggled with hair loss for years before cancer, relying on extensions and other tricks to cover it up. The thought of losing it all was beyond comprehension. I couldn't imagine being "Nic with no hair," or "Mammy without hair" - especially as a hairdresser. It felt like losing a part of my identity. Yet, taking my medication is more important than my hair.

Through all of this, I needed a lifeline. I needed to find someone who *got it*. As much as my family loved me, I didn't want to burden them with my darkest thoughts. My little brother had just become a father, and I didn't want him worrying about me. I realised I needed to connect with others who were living with cancer - people in the same boat as me.

But finding the right group wasn't easy. The worries I faced in my 30s were completely different from what women in their 70s were dealing with. I wanted to talk about fertility, sex, mortgages and running a business - things that didn't come up in every support group. And while many groups were great, some felt like a competition for who had the worst cancer story. If you ever find yourself in one of *those* groups, do yourself a favour – leave.

As a young woman, with a family, running my own business, I didn't know anyone else like me with a cancer diagnosis; I felt so alone. Finding someone like me became vitally important.

I wanted to be in groups that took my mind off cancer yet understood what I was going through. I wanted to be in groups where the people had the same worries as me. I wanted to be in groups where I felt heard and provided opportunities to support other members. "One hand up, one hand down," a wise man once said.

Then, I met Caroline at Shine – a resource for people under 50 with cancer – and she became my lifeline. We shared everything: our fears, our frustrations and the humour we found in it all. We laughed, we cried and we bonded. Caroline and I were a similar age and both loved dressing up and talking about hair, fashion and makeup. She was one of those women whom you admired from afar – always pristine, well-dressed and utterly gorgeous. We could be 100% honest with each other; we saw each other as we were. While she is not here anymore, I'm so very thankful I got to know her because she changed my life for the better and supported me on days when I felt like no one else would understand.

The harsh reality is, that if you do end up finding someone to go through this journey with, you may end up parting ways sooner than you'd wish. Be prepared for that too. Not everyone you meet will get the chance of a cure, but both of your lives will be richer thanks to these connections, no matter how fleeting they may be. Don't let that put you off finding a new community and creating your network.

It didn't matter how much support I had around me, there were times when the only person who could help me was *me*. I had to learn to draw on my own strength, especially when those creeping What Ifs took hold of my mind. A wise psychologist once told me that about 85% of our What Ifs never happen. I clung to that fact.

On the toughest days, I only allowed myself to focus on the next ten minutes. Thinking too far ahead was overwhelming. I treated it like quitting sugar or junk food - just get through the next interval. When the adrenaline hit, I channelled it into movement. I'd go outside, get my heart rate up and breathe in the fresh air. Every little bit helped.

I remind myself that cancer isn't something that just happened to me, it's something I continue to live with every day. Despite being in full remission, in the last eight years, I have attended over 100 doctor and hospital appointments, had four smaller procedures, two major surgeries, eight mammograms, and more than ten MRIs. I'm on meds for the next decade and in a chemically induced menopause. Cancer isn't something you simply have, get over, and forget about. The effects can last a lifetime.

On the flip side, life becomes more vivid, and brighter. It's as if the blinkers have been removed and life becomes this colourful mosaic that you get to piece together, one tiny section at a time. It reminds me of the Japanese practice of Kintsugi, where broken pottery is rendered with gold. We get to take what feels broken, gently bringing it back together, and repairing it with our unique gold.

A life-changing illness like cancer (or indeed any big trauma) makes you appreciate every moment. I no longer worry about getting old - ageing is a privilege that not everyone gets. I, along with millions of others, am proof that you can live with it and after it. You can even thrive, and feel enormous gratitude for each birthday that comes around.

Back to the day that I swore at my husband, when I was feeling truly sorry for myself. As I sat in the hospital waiting room, I took a sudden, deeper notice of something very obvious: There were a lot of bald women in that room with me. In fact, visit after visit, I had noticed woman after woman with her head down, her confidence shattered, her crown gone. I saw bald heads, turbans, and wigs that, in my opinion, looked like wigs rather than natural hair.

As Steve consoled me in that room – a place neither of us wanted to be – I was struck by an epiphany. All the sorrow I had carried through months of treatment began to dissolve. The self-pity, the overwhelm and the endless What Ifs that had consumed me, simply vanished. At that moment, I felt free. I realised my cancer wasn't just about me anymore. It was about what I could do to help others facing their own battles. It was utterly liberating, like handing over the weight of cancer. The burden of focusing on myself shifted, and instead, I embraced a mission bigger than me – a purpose to make a difference in the lives of others. That shift made me feel free in a way I hadn't before.

I can't describe how it felt. My heart rate slowed, the fear lifted and everything seemed brighter, more at peace. It was as if time itself had slowed down. I sat there grinning like an idiot. It was as if somebody tapped me on the shoulder and said, "Nicola, you get it. It's all happening for a reason. This is the reason you've got cancer."

I had spent my whole life making people feel beautiful with their hair but at this moment, I knew I would spend the rest of my days making people feel beautiful without it.

I stopped crying and turned to Steve. I vividly remember telling him I knew why I had cancer. Of course, he gave me that here-we-go look. Considering I'd just been screaming, shouting, and acting like a woman possessed, I don't blame him for wondering what I was rambling on about!

"I know what I need to do. I can help these women without hair and make the process of hair loss easier. Steve, this is why I got cancer – so I can help them feel beautiful too." In that moment, I shifted from "Why me?"

to understanding with perfect clarity and intuition: This is why.

This is the *why.*

The following stories illustrate how cancer is pervasive and affects everyone - the old, the young, sisters, brothers, children, colleagues, mums, and daughters. There's not a single person untouched by it. Even if it feels like you're alone in this journey, you're not. We can all find solace in knowing there's always someone else who understands.

14

The Unexpected Companion

By: Karen Young

Life isn't fair and you can never make sense of cancer or why it chooses you. But I am grateful to have emerged as a survivor. Cancer doesn't discriminate, but neither does the potential for survival.

My journey began in 2015 while my husband and I were living overseas. Back in the UK, my 70-year-old mum was debating whether to have her final mammogram. Thankfully, I was home for the summer, and she decided to go through with it. The results came back, Stage 2 hormonal breast cancer. Shocked and tearful, I took charge, arranging appointments, surgery and radiotherapy. I didn't always know the right thing to say, but I tried to stay positive for her, even when I felt like crumbling inside. I extended my stay in the UK to support her.

Fortunately, Mum didn't need chemotherapy, but the surgery took a toll on her. She had always been so independent, and learning to rely on me wasn't easy for her. Despite her cancer not being genetic, some minor changes in my breast led to my referral for a mammogram. The results were clear, and the doctors reassured me it was highly unlikely that I would develop breast cancer. With Mum's recovery progressing well, my husband and I returned to South America.

In 2016, Nicola, my friend, coworker and yes, the woman behind this book, called to ask about my plans for visiting the UK that summer. I had already planned to return for my mum's one-year checkup. During the conversation, Nicola dropped a bombshell: She had been diagnosed with breast cancer. I was stunned. First my mum, now Nicola.

When I arrived in the UK, a letter awaited me, requesting that I undergo another mammogram. At first, I thought it was a mistake, after all, I'd just had one in 2015 and I was only 48. But then I learned that a trial was being conducted in the Northeast, screening women from age 47 to assess whether lowering the screening age was beneficial. Feeling calm, I went through the process, reassured by last year's clear result. But within 10 days, I received another letter: Something had been detected. I was promptly referred to the Queen Elizabeth Hospital for another mammogram and biopsy. I tried to keep up a light conversation at the appointment, joking about how breast cancer couldn't possibly be in the cards for me. I lived in Colombia, had just rescued a dog and needed to get back to my husband. But beneath that calm exterior, I was more anxious than I cared to admit.

The wait for the next appointment, for which my husband flew back to the UK, felt endless. I still believed it would be nothing. But hearing the diagnosis of Stage 1 hormonal breast cancer was surreal. It was like watching it happen to someone else. The realisation that my mum, Nicola, and now I had all been affected by cancer felt both unbelievable and painfully real.

As I processed the news, I couldn't help but think of my rescue dog, Jago. Who would take care of him? It's funny what your mind clings to in times of crisis.

Navigating the Trials of Treatment

After countless appointments, I had a lumpectomy. I was terrified, thinking things like: Would I come out scarred and unrecognisable? Would my husband still find me attractive? Would I ever feel like myself again? The biggest fear of all was whether I would even survive the surgery. As I regained consciousness afterwards, tears streamed down my face, overwhelmed with relief and gratitude. When they asked if I was okay, I could only cry tears of happiness. I was alive.

I'll never forget the comforting presence of my surgeon, who had also treated both my mum and Nicola. Knowing I was in capable and compassionate hands brought me peace. When I was finally allowed to go home, the joy of seeing my husband, and later my mum and son, was indescribable. The weeks that followed were full of exhaustion and discomfort. My poor husband tirelessly navigated my mood swings, offering support in any way he could.

By early November, it was time for radiotherapy at the Freeman Hospital. It felt like Groundhog Day after going through it with my mum. Cancer knows no boundaries, it affects everyone. I never imagined I'd go from being a supportive companion to a patient myself. But here I was, fighting my own battle. The daily routine of radiotherapy for 15 consecutive days can take a toll on your spirit. While the treatment itself is brief once you're positioned, the process of getting there, waiting and enduring the treatment is a mental and emotional marathon. By the second week, I was sore, a side effect I hadn't expected. On the 15th day, I rang the bell. It felt strange to be done, knowing I wouldn't see the familiar faces again, but I was relieved to have finished.

Now, my challenge was to get fit enough to return to my husband and our rescue dog, Jago, in Colombia as my body was getting used to Tamoxifen.

Finding Strength Together

Throughout this journey, the solidarity I found in my mum and Nicola was invaluable. We had all battled breast cancer within a year of each other, and that shared experience gave me a sense of companionship in an otherwise isolating journey. Through it all, I worked hard to maintain normality and resilience, refusing to let cancer make me feel like a victim.

It's so important to listen to your body and honour its needs. Whether that means resting or staying active, you must prioritise what feels right for you. And if you're reading this after a cancer diagnosis, know that it's okay to feel angry or emotional. Help is available.

Talking helps. With over 40 years of experience as a hairdresser, I had the privilege of meeting countless individuals. After my battle with cancer, my career took a new direction.

In 2018, I joined Nicola as a Medical Hair Loss Consultant. Becoming part of the Cancer Club means I have the privilege of helping thousands of people navigate the trauma of hair loss with our team at The Wonderful Wig Company. Wearing a wig can feel scary if you've never tried one before, but with guidance, the process becomes easier. We offer options that look incredibly natural, from synthetic to human hair wigs. Seeing our clients regain their confidence is priceless. It's transformed my cancer journey into something deeply meaningful and positive.

I'll never forget one Christmas when a client told my husband that, aside from the medical professionals who saved her life, I had the most significant impact on her cancer journey. Hearing that filled him with immense pride.

My husband often refers to me as a survivor, and I've come to embrace that label. Life holds deeper meaning now, and while I still have moments of post-cancer blues, I've accepted them as a normal part of this process, a reminder to keep moving forward.

15

Living Strong

By Brenda Lofthouse and Sarah Pavlou

Sarah:

I'll never forget the moment I got the news. I was on holiday, visiting my husband's family in Cyprus when my world flipped upside down. For months, mum had been dealing with what she thought was a reaction to coffee or irritable bowel syndrome. But after an investigation into her bowel, they found a tumour.

At first, I was in denial, thinking, How could this be happening? No one in our family had ever had cancer. It felt like a mistake. But four hours later, it hit me like a tidal wave. A deep sense of loss and overwhelming emotion took over, and I broke down. Mum is my best friend and I wasn't ready to lose her.

But Mum? She was as strong as ever. "I have cancer," she said, "but it's treatable, and the doctors are amazing at what they can do these days. I won't let it beat me. Let's see what the doctors say." Right from the start, her determination to keep living a normal life was undeniable. She wasn't just fighting cancer; she was defying it.

Brenda:

I couldn't believe it at first. There's no history of cancer in our family, and I've always been healthy. I quit smoking over fifty years ago, and kept active by walking the hills. "How could this be real?" I thought.

Then it hit me: I'm human, after all. There's an element of fate in life, and sometimes, no matter how hard you try, things just happen. I accepted it. This was my reality now. But I wasn't angry or afraid, there were so many people around me who had beaten cancer or were still fighting it. Cancer didn't have to be a death sentence. With the right attitude, I knew I could face it, just like I'd faced other challenges in my life.

Sarah:

I kept asking Mum how she felt, but her answer was always the same: "I'm fine." Her goal had always been to outlive her mother, who passed away at 93, and to be at my son's 21st and 18th birthday parties. "I have a mission, and I will fulfil it," she'd say.

Mum often remarked, "Despite being 81, no one in the NHS ever made me feel like I wasn't worth saving."

Overcoming Mum's Challenges

Sarah:

Getting Mum into chemotherapy took longer than we expected. What started as bowel cancer spread slightly to her liver, changing her treatment plan. Initially, surgery was on the table, followed by chemo. But with the liver involvement, the approach became non-curative, with the doctors focusing on her liver first. They worried that surgery, at 81, would be too risky for her.

Eating became painful for Mum, and soon, her bowel was at risk of exploding. The hospital had to fit a stent to open it up, allowing things to pass. That helped, but her diet became so limited, and her weight started to fall off.

Her chemo began with a three-hour drip at the hospital, followed by two weeks of pills. For the first four days, she felt fine, strong, like herself. But then everything changed. She was bedridden, no energy, barely eating. A week later, she found a lump in her abdomen, it was a hernia, so we rushed her to the hospital. Luckily, the hernia wasn't strangulated, so no surgery was needed. But when her oncologist saw how weak she had become, he decided to change her treatment plan. A Hickman line was inserted, and her chemo switched to a 46-hour slow drip, followed by a 12-day break. That gave her a chance to rebuild her strength.

But during the waiting period, Mum's breathing worsened. The hospital found small clots in her lungs, manageable for now, but concerning. She started blood thinners, and eventually, we got everything under control. When her second round of chemo finally began, it was much easier on her. She felt tired, yes, but she could live her life again.

How We Coped Together

Sarah:

After the second round of chemo, Mum's hair began falling out. It was time to shave the rest and embrace a wig. But true to form, she took it all in stride, saying, "It's just hair; it will grow back." I took her to Nicola's The Wonderful Wig Company where I knew the experience would be more like a treat than something to dread. The entire process, from the warm greeting to the follow-up email, was full of empathy, fun and care. In a dark time, it was a moment of light, and Mum left feeling like her beautiful self again.

Brenda:

My hair has always been important to me. It's what made me feel good, and sometimes, not so good. Even though I knew it would grow back, losing it was hard. But at The Wonderful Wig Company, I felt so special, so cared for. The wig I have now feels like mine. When I look in the mirror, I see the real me.

The hats are handy at home or when it's cold, but the wig? That's my preference. It helps me maintain a sense of normality, which is crucial when facing something as daunting as cancer. My earrings and makeup play a big role too. Every day, I remind myself: I'm still here, I'm alive, and I'm living.

I believe it is important to share my own experiences and highlight the many services in just my local area. I hope to help others find the same faith and determination to overcome cancer.

Sarah:

It was interesting to see how my brother and dad responded as Mum began to manage her chemo. My brother became obsessed with finding the right foods to help her digestion. My dad, on the other hand, wanted to keep Mum home, away from any potential illnesses. He focused on making sure she was warm and rested, keeping everything as private as possible.

Brenda:

Having to rely on others was the hardest part for me. It felt like a complete role reversal and one I hadn't expected. My son lives in Leeds, so he helped from a distance, while Sarah, who lives nearby, supported me every day.

Sarah:

I took on the responsibility of making the whole experience as comfortable as possible for Mum. I knew she would worry about everyone else but herself, so I made sure meals were ready, the house was stocked with food and the washing was done.

Brenda:

The support from the hospital staff was a huge source of strength. Friends and family who visited or called kept me going. When I felt down, I reached out. One of my best friends, who had passed away two years earlier, had a son who'd been battling cancer for four years. He was a big support because he understood what it felt like.

Here's What We Learned

Sarah:

It's okay to feel strange emotions, and it's okay to take care of yourself too. As people kept telling me, "Be kind to yourself, Sarah."

Brenda:

You don't need to bombard people with all the details, but it's important to talk. Be honest about how you feel, and don't be afraid to ask for help. When family members fussed over tasks I used to handle easily, it frustrated me. But as I stayed as active and mobile as possible, I regained control over my life and that gave me strength, both mentally and physically.

16

Making Tough Decisions

Anonymous

My second child had been a grumbly baby from the start, never too keen on feeding. It was New Year's Eve, 1996, when my gut instinct kicked in, it was time to check in with the GP. My little one hadn't fed for three days.

Exhausted and juggling my 21-month-old clinging to my leg, I sat in front of the doctor. She asked how long my three-month-old had had a temperature. I felt awful, I hadn't even noticed in my sleep-deprived haze. Before I knew it, we were in A&E, my baby wobbling on a cardboard kidney bowl for five hours while we desperately tried to get a tiny wee out of their dehydrated body.

The New Year was spent in an isolation room, my baby hooked up to intravenous fluids and antibiotics, battling what turned out to be a severe urinary infection. Somehow, amidst the chaos, the nurses snuck a bottle of fizz into the medication fridge, and we had a quick five-minute party to welcome in 1997.

Further tests revealed something troubling. The consultant noticed a wavy edge on their left kidney, growing at an alarming rate. He suspected cancer and sent everything to Great Ormond Street Children's Hospital for analysis. The experts initially thought it was just a cyst, but our consultant wasn't convinced. More scans showed the mass was growing fast, and off we went to London.

It wasn't long before we got the diagnosis: a Wilms tumour, common in children but needing prompt removal. My baby was only eight months old when they underwent a lengthy operation. The surgeon managed to remove both the tumour and the kidney, which had been engulfed by the growth.

We were told to go home and enjoy our baby.

But just five months later, at a check-up, the cancer had returned. Another surgery, another gruelling battle. This time, the surgeon removed a mass he described as "raw fish flesh," unlike anything he'd seen. It turned out to be a rare, previously incurable form of kidney cancer. Suddenly, survival was a coin toss, a terrifying 50/50.

My little one, now with huge scars and puckered skin from the lines inserted into their body, was utterly dependent on me. It felt like the weight of the world rested on my shoulders.

One morning, sitting in the kitchen with a cup of tea, I made three decisions: first, I had to keep my baby alive, making the best possible choices for their care; second, I needed to ensure my eldest, only three, was well looked after so they weren't overshadowed by their sibling's illness; and third, somehow, I had to hold the family together and get us all through this.

So, I girded my loins and f*cking got on with it.

Making Sh*t Happen

I became an expert in quick decisions, knowing when my child needed urgent hospital care and when I could push to get them home earlier so they could play with their sibling. I trusted my gut, my decisions and my ability to fight for them because I had no other choice.

The team at Great Ormond Street introduced a trial chemo protocol, a toxic cocktail dropped straight into my child's heart. Nurses warned that if it spilt, it would burn a hole through the lino! We spent months in and out of the hospital and then came seven weeks of daily radiotherapy, which meant waking at 6 am to drive to London every day.

My little one barely ate during those long days. Maybe I'd get one Dolly Mixture into their mouth while we watched *Spot the Dog* on repeat. Their older sibling, however, devoured every meal, growing into a bouncing preschooler while my baby grew frailer. By the end of treatment, they had no hair, no eyelashes, and no eyebrows. Their bum sagged; their stomach distended – it broke my heart.

Through it all, my child's resilience amazed me. They loved showing off their "Snakey" (the Hickman line) whenever the doctors asked if they wanted a milky drink, pulling it out with a proud little nod. Post-chemo, watching them ram in a "jam sammidge" at high speed, was a tiny, joyful victory.

Surrounded By Support and Love

My now ex-husband's family was an incredible support system, despite living over 100 miles away. They spoiled my eldest while doting on my youngest. My mother-in-law, Nanny, always found fun activities to brighten their day.

The local churches put us on their prayer lists, and I'll never forget how comforting that was. It felt like a warm pashmina of love wrapped around me, holding us all together. Friends would call while they were at the supermarket, offering to pick up milk or bread when my foggy mind couldn't keep track of the basics. Some friends even took turns doing our laundry, handing it back to me neatly pressed, an impossible luxury at the time.

When I had a moment to breathe, I'd steal away for pizza with my girlfriends, a good laugh, a needed cry or even a healing Reiki session.

Unforeseen Challenges

In 2007, when my youngest was 12 and we were living elsewhere in Europe, they suddenly fell ill. One night, after coming home from their dad's, I noticed their normally skinny legs were swollen to the size of an elephant's. We rushed to the hospital, where they were diagnosed with serious heart failure.

It turned out that the chemotherapy had damaged their heart beyond repair, and they also had a large clot in their heart. A week later, my baby suffered a massive stroke, leaving them with right-side hemiplegia (paralysis) and in urgent need of a heart transplant.

The fight to get them back to the UK was brutal. With life-saving drugs pumping into their heart 24/7 via a battery, airlines refused to let us fly. But I wasn't about to give up. With help from some wonderful pilots, we were flown back to England, first class.

After a long journey of recovery, osteopathy, and many tears, my child finally received a new heart. Their resilience was nothing short of a miracle. But the years that followed were filled with new struggles of anxiety, depression, and addiction as they tried to navigate adulthood with the weight of everything they'd been through.

Guidance for Long-Haul Support

For anyone in a support role, know this: You're in it for the long haul, so you'll have to toughen up and just get on with it. Life's not about fairness, it's about getting through the storms and learning from them. You're stronger than you think, and you'll find that strength in ways you never imagined.

I look back and I know I acted in the best interests of my child at each point of their journey. Sometimes I had to fight to get them the care I knew they needed and I would do it all again, in a heartbeat.

With every tough decision I made, I reminded myself of the grit that had gotten me this far. I seem to have passed that determination on to my youngest.

When the advice of doctors clashed with my gut, I trusted myself. You should too. Because when you're in the darkest of places, failure simply isn't an option.

17

Small Changes, Big Impact

By Caroline Tweedie

As a Clinical Breast Nurse Specialist since 2006, I've had the privilege of supporting hundreds of women (and men) and their families through their cancer journeys. For many, receiving a cancer diagnosis is like having their world implode. The initial emotions vary from shock and fear to sadness, anger, and disbelief. Some people experience these emotions all at once, while others move through them in waves.

Cancer treatment is deeply personal, and no two experiences are the same. It depends on the type and stage of cancer, overall health, and the patient's preferences. Milestones like completing surgery, finishing chemotherapy, or achieving remission bring a sense of progress, but the challenges don't stop there. Managing side effects, facing emotional turmoil, and handling complications all add layers of complexity to the journey.

Daily routines often go out the window as treatment demands frequent hospital visits, tests, and managing side effects. Relationships can become strained due to the emotional burden, and caregivers, while vital, may also experience stress.

Work, social life, and daily activities get disrupted too, and adjusting to this new reality often means making sacrifices, whether of time, energy, or even financial resources.

Throughout my time as a Breast CNS, I've also specialised in health and well-being, qualifying as a personal trainer and cancer rehab practitioner. I've learned that small, incremental changes in lifestyle can go a long way in helping patients through treatment and recovery.

The Power of Small Changes

Simple lifestyle changes, like improving diet, increasing exercise and practising self-care can significantly enhance quality of life during and after treatment. Emotional and psychological well-being also play a huge role in recovery. It's these small, seemingly minor adjustments that often make the biggest impact on the overall journey.

Each person's experience with cancer is unique, and the way it affects daily life varies. This is why the support of healthcare professionals, family and friends is so crucial. Specialist Breast Care Nurses provide emotional support, education and practical help. We're trained to recognise moments of crisis and respond with immediate support to help individuals navigate the mental and emotional challenges of cancer.

Some patients have described a diagnosis like receiving a grenade, others see it as a wake-up call that leads to a more intentional, fulfilling life. I've seen women reframe their priorities by choosing to live in the moment, invest in daily joy and rethink long-term plans.

Lessons from Years of Experience

One thing I've learned is the importance of open, honest communication with loved ones. Sometimes, people are afraid of saying the wrong thing, so they say nothing at all. Don't assume others don't care if they haven't been in touch, they might just be unsure how to approach you.

Surround yourself with those who lift you up, "radiators" as I call them, and keep those who drain your energy at a distance when you're feeling low. Your support system is essential, and asking for help when you need it is a sign of strength, not weakness.

If your emotional reserves are running low, seek professional support, whether through counselling, support groups or mental health services. One of the best treatments for breast cancer patients? Regular movement. Even gentle exercise can help rebuild self-confidence, improve mood, and reduce anxiety. It can even improve sleep and reduce the symptoms of mild depression.

There's also evidence that regular physical activity can reduce the risk of cancer recurrence. Women who maintained regular activity both before and after diagnosis were less likely to have their cancer return or experience complications. If your doctor approves, even light exercise like walking, yoga, or stretching can be beneficial during treatment. Start slow, listen to your body and gradually increase your activity.

Inspiration from Patients

Cancer patients never cease to inspire me. Their resilience, courage, and determination have been the reason I've stayed in cancer care for so long. Despite the toll cancer takes, I've witnessed countless individuals find joy, laughter, and gratitude in the smallest moments, reminding us all to appreciate life even in the hardest times.

Experiencing the vulnerability of illness often develops a deep sense of empathy and compassion. Their ability to connect with others on an emotional level can inspire those around them to cultivate greater understanding and kindness. This is why I involve those with lived experience when I offer group sessions, as they can offer so much expertise.

The transformative nature of a cancer diagnosis often leads to profound personal growth. Cancer patients may inspire others to view challenges as opportunities for self-discovery and personal development.

When Small Changes Matter Most

One patient who was struggling with Tamoxifen was terrified to take it because of the side effects but equally scared of the consequence of not taking it in case her cancer returned (a widespread concern). She had previously tried the medication but found the menopausal side effects very debilitating and made it clear she couldn't continue and decided she wanted to know the alternatives. I referred her to the oncologist to discuss her options; however, while she waited for this consultation, I wanted her to start increasing her daily activity, reduce her alcohol intake, and work towards a healthy BMI.

I explained the increased protection she would get from embracing a healthier lifestyle; unfortunately, she took this advice personally, burst into tears, walked out of the consultation, and slammed the door. I tried to ring her and offer her support, but she refused to answer my calls. I made another appointment, and she failed to attend; eventually, after two months, she returned to the clinic.

She looked remarkably different, and she had this most fantastic smile. She started the consultation by apologising for her behaviour; she said she had left the initial consultation distraught and went straight to the off-licence, bought two bottles of Prosecco, a tub of Pringles, and a family-size bar of dairy milk chocolate, and ate and drank the lot in one sitting.

The next day, she woke and looked in the mirror, and she realised that something had to change. She decided to have a dry February and committed to moving more, getting off two stops earlier on her bus journey to work. It was truly inspiring to see her keep an open mind to my advice, even when taking those first steps towards change felt challenging.

After a few weeks, she got rid of her bus pass and walked the whole journey. She started slowly tweaking her diet, cutting out the crisps and chocolate but continuing to have a once-weekly takeaway as a treat. Her lifestyle has transformed her wardrobe; losing two stones has changed her shape and allowed her to buy the dream outfit she wanted for her son's wedding. The aches and pains have slowly been replaced with a new sense of energy, and finally, she was getting consistent sleep.

She thanked me for being brave and tackling the elephant in the room and feels she has finally got her silver lining from her breast cancer diagnosis. Of course, encouraging patients to make positive changes in their lives is part of the job, but it's especially rewarding when it leads to a silver lining like this.

Final Thoughts

I am incredibly fortunate to witness the strength, courage, and resilience of cancer patients every day. Their journeys serve as powerful reminders of the strength of the human spirit and the capacity to find inspiration, even in the face of adversity.

18

No One Size Fits All

By Sarah Pittendrigh

Raising awareness about skin cancer has become one of my main focuses, especially through social media. I try to contribute in various ways whether it's participating in charity events like the Mighty Hike for Macmillan or hosting Macmillan Coffee Mornings. But my connection to this cause is personal. I've been diagnosed with malignant melanoma twice, and both times, I faced it head-on.

In 2015, a routine trip to an aesthetics clinic with my mum turned into a life-changing moment. During a facial, the practitioner, who happened to specialise in skin cancer, noticed a suspicious mole on the side of my head. It was bleeding, which is never a good sign. I booked an appointment with a surgeon at Jesmond Nuffield Hospital, and the mole was promptly removed. The news came back: malignant melanoma.

A second surgery followed to ensure all cancerous cells were excised, which was a relief, but the experience left its mark. Then, in 2016, I was diagnosed again, this time with a mole on my chest. The process was all too familiar: surgery, follow-ups and that same waiting for test results. Fortunately, I've been cancer-free since, but I remain vigilant, attending annual check-ups. Over the years, I've had 14 moles removed – thankfully all benign.

You'd think catching it early would erase the fear, but it doesn't. Facing cancer, even early-stage, demands every bit of your courage. Every procedure, every surgery, is a test of resilience. It's a strange thing, realising that even when you beat the odds, the mental scars run deep. You carry them long after the physical ones fade.

Now, sunbathing is a distant memory. I'm always covered up, wearing factor 50 sunscreen. I allow myself just enough sun to avoid burning and ensure I get my daily dose of vitamin D, which is important as I approach midlife and face concerns like osteoporosis. But no more tanning for me.

My family and specialists have been my support network throughout these times. They helped me navigate the confusion, especially in the beginning when I feared the cancer might spread.

Regardless of the type of cancer, that uncertainty always lingers. You start scrutinising every change in your body. You ask yourself again and again, "What if it's back? What if I missed something?"

One of the hardest lessons I learned was to stop Googling symptoms. It's so easy to spiral when you're faced with the unknown. But cancer is a personal journey. It's critical to remember that no two cases are the same. Don't let the internet decide your fate. Only take advice from your specialists because your case is unique, and only they can guide you through it.

Leaning on others who've walked a similar path can be invaluable. They get it – the rollercoaster of emotions, the fear, the relief, and everything in between. But even then, it's important to remember that their journey isn't yours. There's no "right" way to cope with cancer. Each of us deals with it differently, and that's okay. It's your story, and no one else's.

I'll never forget what a friend once said to me, though: "You haven't really had cancer, not proper cancer," just because I hadn't gone through chemotherapy. It hurt deeply and made me feel like a fraud as if my experience wasn't valid. For a while, I kept my diagnosis quiet because of that. But here's the thing: No one has the right to tell you how to feel about your diagnosis. Whether you've had chemo or not, surgery or not, your experience is real, and your emotions are valid. Never let someone else's ignorance undermine your journey.

Instead of letting hurtful comments affect you, use them as a catalyst for education. Challenge them to learn more, to understand before they speak. In doing so, you shift the conversation to something constructive: awareness and empathy. We can all benefit from a little more of that.

As I learned, don't be afraid to ask questions. If something feels off, talk to your consultant. If you're anxious, share it. You don't have to be superhuman. You need your energy to focus on getting better. Lean on those around you for support, and most importantly, live for the now. Cancer teaches you this more than anything else: Tomorrow isn't guaranteed. Yesterday is behind us. All we have is today.

19

A Son's Perspective on

Cancer in the Family

By Gabriel Wood, Age 14

It happened when I was six years old. My mam (or my mammy back then) and dad called for me, and she said she wanted to speak with me. I went in, jumped up on her lap and cuddled her. She then read me a book about cancer and explained to me that she had been diagnosed with it.

I was very scared and quite confused because I was only six and I did not know what cancer was or what it did. "Was my mam going to die?" I thought back then cancer only killed people. It was very upsetting seeing my mam cry, but she explained she might get a little sad sometimes too. I didn't get it. All I knew was my mam and dad had said it was going to be okay, so in my mind that was all I needed to know.

The next thing I remember was my mam and dad going to the hospital every single day. It was in the six weeks of school holidays, and I remember going to the hospital when all I wanted to do was play and have fun. We used to have to leave the house at 8am. I just remember that we were all touring the hospital every morning. We were not there too long each day.

I was always allowed some sweets and at the time I was really into a Pokémon game; normally I wasn't allowed on the phone too much, but I was allowed to play it every day at the hospital – result! I just used to run around the grounds of the hospital looking for Pokémons on my mam's phone. There were so many cool and unusual Pokémon while I was there, and they all kept me occupied. I loved it.

Looking back, I didn't realise what cancer was. I was quite confused as to why we were going off to the hospital every day. On some days, I recall thinking that my parents were doing some work in a hospital, then other days I'd remember, that my mam was quite poorly, and it was sad to see her like that. Other days she was in so much pain, but I didn't really know what was going on. As long as she kept telling me everything was okay, I knew it would be.

Mam's Reassuring Hugs

My parents were really good at making everything feel okay. They made me feel safe. When my mam stayed home instead of going to work, I got to spend more time with her. That meant extra cuddles, which made everything feel a lot better. In my six-year-old mind, it didn't seem so bad. To me, those cuddles meant everything was okay and mam would be alright.

Knowing about my mam's cancer diagnosis made things better. If I hadn't known, and she just went to the hospital every day, I think I would have been a lot more worried. But because I knew what was happening, I could understand it a bit more. That's why I think it's important to be honest with your family, even the younger ones. Kids are observant and unexplained changes in routine can create a lot of confusion. Just tell us the truth, and maybe we can even help in our way.

If I hadn't known and found out later, I think I would have been a lot more upset. Weirdly, knowing about it early on made things a lot easier because it allowed me to process it. Open communication, even though it was difficult, made the whole situation a lot more manageable.

The hospital visits felt easier because I had a big distraction: my phone. I was glued to it the whole time. As silly as it sounds, it helped me a lot to just not think about what was happening. At home, having my parents with me more was comforting. Usually, they're at work during the day, so seeing them more and spending extra time together felt good.

Looking back, I realise that even though the distractions helped, what really made things easier was knowing the truth. My parents were always open with me, which made a huge difference.

Keeping It Real

My best advice for cancer patients who have children is to tell them right away. It's important not to keep it a secret, as that could make it seem scarier for them. Being open helps the child understand what's happening and will prevent them from getting upset if they eventually find out or if the situation changes. Cancer will continue to affect your family's life, long after the initial diagnosis so it should not be a secret.

To all the kids out there, my wish for you is to learn how not to let cancer interfere with your life. Keep living as you always have but remember to acknowledge its presence and offer support to your loved one in any way you can. Even a small gesture on a bad day can make them feel a million times better.

I think the long-lasting impact of someone you know going through cancer is that not every hospital trip or doctor's visit is directly related to cancer. I would worry every time someone, especially my mam, was sick. I guess that's normal for a while I would always think, "Has something happened?" It took me some time to grasp that cancer was no longer the dominant force in our lives.

As a child, I saw a lot of stories on TV of people losing their battle with cancer, which made me think it always ended badly. But as I grew older and saw my mam not only survive but thrive after her diagnosis, I began to understand that cancer isn't always fatal. This realisation completely changed how I viewed her illness. Instead of constantly fearing the worst, I learned to focus on the present and the good moments we had together. It gave me a new sense of hope and helped me stop worrying as much. Knowing that people can live with and overcome cancer made me feel more positive, not just about her journey, but about life in general.

How Cancer Became Our Unlikely Inspiration

My mam having cancer was not great at the start. It was upsetting of course, but it's been probably the biggest positive thing in our entire lives, and it's changed the way we look at things.

Cancer even changed my mam's entire field of work. She used to be a hairdresser and now she works with cancer patients every day. She's winning awards for helping people and as much as cancer is a bad thing, it makes me proud to see how my mam's adapted it and used it to help people with her own experience.

I believe the message is that even though cancer is terrible and can affect anyone, it changes how we perceive things. Over the past six or seven years, our lives have evolved, giving us a different perspective. Our family has grown closer as a result. I am grateful for my parents' honesty with me and for trusting me with the truth. I now have a better understanding of what my mam has been through, and I can help her better.

20

Reflections by a Consultant Clinical Psychologist

By Dr. Peter Blackburn

The aim of this reflection is to illustrate that while most people I meet with cancer tell a similar story, it is also unique because it is their personal story. I hope that this reflection can show that you are not alone.

On meeting a patient, who is being treated, or has completed cancer treatment, they tell a familiar story about diagnosis and what has happened to them afterwards. It is familiar because I have heard a variation of it many times but it is also unique.

Before people get cancer, they are going about their lives in their usual way with hopes, dreams, regrets, concerns, fears and worries, and then their lives change dramatically following a diagnosis of cancer. Their lives are turned upside down because they have either found some sign or symptom of cancer, this may be a lump or blood or they've gone for a routine investigation or routine surveillance, such as a mammogram, and something is found.

Then what often happens, but not always, something suspicious is taken seriously and the person is on a pathway to being investigated more fully. These investigations are often uncomfortable, and intrusive and test a person's sense of dignity.

The diagnostic process often happens very quickly and that can be a big shock. For others, they may have had their suspicions and it's not such a big shock.

The next step is that the person enters a treatment pathway, which has been likened to a conveyor belt, a rollercoaster, or a merry-go-round. At this stage, things are happening to the person that tests and challenges them physically, mentally, and socially.

When people get to the end of treatment, they may be pleased to ring the bell, or they may not, because it does not feel like good news to them or the end. The good news means that the medical teams can step back as they are no longer needed.

Often the family and friends step back too because they hear the good news and conclude they are no longer needed for support. This stepping back is often too quick for the person who has been through treatment, and they can feel abandoned. However, for some, it's just the end of the first half of what this new life is about, because the second half is trying to make sense - both intellectually but more so emotionally - of what they have been through and who they are now, with a future that feels less certain.

A person's experience of being diagnosed and treated for cancer can be very quick, which can be a huge relief. It can also be traumatic because they are unable to process what has and is happening; but also because of the nature of the threat. A few people will have symptoms that would reach a diagnosis of post-traumatic stress disorder (PTSD) but for many more people, they have some of the symptoms of PTSD.

Either way, these symptoms can be awful and disruptive. If they experience such symptoms, then they can discuss these with their GP. Often it is only when people feel safe that they start to experience trauma symptoms, which can be confusing because they feel they should be happy.

Most people can make sense of traumatic experiences if they can talk to friends and family whom they trust and who are good listeners. Some people need professional help to process their experiences.

The same can be true for a sense of grief for the changes that have occurred. Some people find it hard to understand that they are grieving because nobody has died. However, significant loss can lead to profound feelings of sorrow and anger. As with symptoms of trauma, if they can talk through the emotional pain associated with loss with trusted others who just listen (rather than try to fix it), then this can be very helpful. Other approaches to loss that can be helpful are writing about experiences or speaking to a professional.

Please don't forget that you are not alone in what you are thinking and feeling. Most people's thoughts and feelings are understandable given what they have or are going through. The diagnosis of cancer and subsequent treatment can have a profound effect on a person's wellbeing, in a variety of ways: physical, psychological, emotional, socio-economic, and spiritual. It is hoped that no one suffers and that timely support can be found for all.

Reflections from Nicola

Cancer doesn't discriminate by age or circumstance. It reminds us that the same illness that strikes our loved ones may find its way into our own lives. Embracing each challenge with resilience is key.

Maintaining normality and a positive attitude, even during the hardest times, can strengthen both the patient and the family. Sometimes, the key to surviving cancer is continuing to live life on your own terms. As a caregiver, trusting your instincts and making tough decisions is essential. Being present and proactive for your loved one makes all the difference, especially when the road is long and uncertain.

Small lifestyle changes, like increasing daily activity and improving diet, can have a massive impact on recovery and quality of life. It's about embracing what's within your control during uncertain times. Each cancer journey is deeply personal and unique. It's important to honour your own experience and not compare it to others. Every diagnosis is valid, no matter the treatment or outcome.

Honest communication, even with children, provides clarity and comfort during difficult times. Open dialogue allows families to face challenges together, making the journey more manageable for everyone.

Cancer not only affects the body but also profoundly impacts the mind and emotions, often leaving patients feeling as though they're on a rollercoaster. The trauma and grief that accompany a cancer diagnosis need to be acknowledged and processed, whether through trusted conversations or professional help. It's important to understand that these feelings are normal, and seeking support is key to healing, both during and after treatment.

Chapter 4
Hair, Healing, and Hope

When I was 12, I got my first Saturday job in a busy salt-of-the-earth style salon in one of the roughest parts of the city. I was on my feet 10 hours a day shampooing, sweeping, taking coats, emptying ashtrays, being shouted at from all directions and rarely getting a lunch break. The pay was £10 for the day but the tips were good. The people were kind and genuinely interested in me. I felt valued and I bloody loved it.

The stylists were amazing. They could blow dry at the speed of light, charging £8 a time, as the relentless, steady stream of regular weekly clients all with the same style came in through the door. "Beans on Toast" we juniors called the signature cut, with its short back and sides, and one inch left on the top which would be tightly permed - a style that required maintenance every week. *Ching ching*. Within 20 minutes of entering the salon, a client was washed, trimmed, had a fag with the stylist, had a coffee and was finished with a blow dry. It was class and I was hooked on hairdressing for the rest of my life.

From there I worked my way up the ladder at Saks. It was posh, upmarket, in the town centre and expensive. Some of the clientele were on the stuck-up side. The tips were crap; I felt invisible there and definitely not appreciated by the clients. I mastered my art, but I learned a valuable lesson in resilience. It also gave me the grit and determination I needed to excel at hair.

I eventually settled at a place just perfect for me – Monets. And under the guidance of my mentor Karen Young (who also shares her story here) and her team, I learned my craft, was appreciated and progressed quickly into a confident talented stylist.

When I was first diagnosed with cancer and hiding myself away at home in a cupboard, brushing away my fears of death and hair loss, I'd never have believed that I'd have this dream. I would never have imagined that I'd suddenly feel alive again because of my cancer.

It was so clear when my epiphany to make women feel beautiful by making better wigs struck me like a lightning bolt in the hospital waiting room – after I'd finished my hysterical rant with Steve – I knew I had what it would take to make this happen. After all, when it comes to hair, I was more than confident.

I had a purpose and a dream. It was so clear: none of my clients who ever lost their hair would have a shitty hair-loss experience. They would have support because I'd make sure they would have alternative hair that didn't look like a wig. No client of mine would ever wear one of those awful wigs I'd seen enter the hospital waiting room so many times, making the woman wearing it lower her head with shame, praying nobody would catch her eye and give her a knowing glance. They would never feel embarrassed. Regardless of their diagnosis, I would make sure they always felt beautiful.

Those days I'd spent trying to make time speed up while I sat in that cold, clinical waiting room between appointments and treatment, watching women shuffle shamefully in trying not to draw attention to their bald heads, their turbans, or their wigs that looked like wigs, were all meant to be. All of those passing comments I'd regularly made to my husband with my hairdresser's head on saying stuff like: "Wow, you'd think wigs would have gotten a bit better by now, wouldn't you?" And "Wow, I wish I could give her wig a cut and style."

They were all leading me to this point: **my purpose**.

I had the bit between my teeth. I had a light burning bright inside of me and forgot about the "thing" that might still be fighting to grow and floor me again. I was excited and of course, being who I was, I became a tad obsessed. But at least I wasn't obsessing over my cancer.

There was question after question, thought after thought, idea after idea in my buzzing head. I felt like I was alive, back in the world of the living.

During my recovery, I started to do research and looked at how to train in hair loss. I got my husband on board, and we'd travel across the country to find the best and worst services in England. I needed to know it all. I researched what support was out there: what wigs and hair alternatives were available, what it was like when you went for a consultation, what the rooms were like, what the wigs and prices were like, what training went into the service and anything else that I unearthed along the way. Then I went deeper. I asked questions like: Why was there such a stigma about wigs? Why was there such a stigma about hair loss? Why was no one who worked in hair loss under 40 years of age?

As a hairdresser, I saw hair as fashion and art. It moves with time. The hair loss industry on the other hand, that one was taboo. If you went in for a consultation, the usual service involved you going into a secluded area with doors locked behind you or curtains drawn, enveloping you to hide you away. The message was clear: You should feel ashamed of your hair loss. I wanted to bring some normality to this experience.

It used to drive me crazy that you'd have to go to the bloody hospital to get your wig. Here, people with no experience with hair were giving you hair advice! It was astounding to me. I could see space for huge improvements at the service level. The excitement burned brighter, and so did the anger at how women were being made to feel.

As I began to understand more about the process and got more and more emotional about the current services available, I knew I wanted to tackle a bigger issue: Educating people about hair loss and letting them know, those in the medical profession included, that this is not about vanity.

Hair loss is not a cosmetic issue. It is a medical one.

When I was first diagnosed, I had two questions. First, "Am I going to die?" and second, "Am I going to lose my hair?" The importance of this second question has become my guiding light. Maybe it was the hairdresser in me, maybe it was the woman in me, or as I know now, it was simply the human in me. My whole perspective on hair and life changed as I asked that question.

For most women, hair loss is their main concern when they are told they have cancer and will require chemotherapy as part of their treatment. There is nothing cosmetic or vain about it. Cancer eats away at your self-worth and hair loss is a public sign that you have it. The label you've been doing your best to hide from to avoid the stares, the pity and the questions is now available for everyone to see. It takes away your power of choice.

I decided to disrupt this industry and turn it on its head.

I set my sights on extending our salon to build a beautiful private space for people with hair loss. It took loads of money but I played the cancer card to my husband and we borrowed some from my lovely father-in-law, Harry, to make it possible. We were skint at the time; cancer has that effect too. I hadn't worked for months and I'd needed to borrow money to keep my business going while I was off! Initially, Steve had looked at me like I was crazy, but then he agreed to my grand plans and set off to work tirelessly night and day for a year to build the extension we needed. They do say love is blind.

We would not lock doors in back rooms for our consultations. Not a single wig or weird mannequin head would be on show. The women would walk into the front door with their heads held high. If they wanted to sit with every other single client in there, they could. If they wanted to come in hooked up to a drip, that was fine. We would hold their hands before they lost all their hair, as they lost it, and after. We would create an inclusive and exclusive atmosphere for our customers, where both those with and without hair would feel beautiful, serviced, and supported.

Next came the wigs. Day and night I researched and developed my ideas. Constantly brainstorming and note scribbling. I completed as many courses as I could and then some. I wanted to ensure that I covered the whole journey - before, during and after hair loss. I wanted to know all of the options that were available and which suppliers we could use. As an independent company, we could source wigs from all over the world. Some wig shops may have 300 pieces to choose from, but we have nearly 30,000 options that we can access.

I wanted to be at the top of my game, so I pushed for the best training courses and scoured the internet for the right information to make sure I knew it all. I also wanted to support nurses with up-to-date information as I'd seen how many facts were outdated and there was such disparity in the information given to people across the country. It riled me that women were being told the wrong information on top of being given an unnatural-looking wig, or maybe no wig at all.

I was ready to go. I was informed, skilled, equipped and the doors were opened. It was time to make it happen. In the sanctuary that my husband had built, I decided to start filming videos for our new services. I set it up, took a few clips and uploaded them to the internet. I felt very vulnerable doing it, but I saw it as my way to support people and raise awareness.

The old Nicola was beginning to emerge. My confidence, determination, grit and energy – the traits that had always made me want to make things happen enabled me to put my face in front of the camera, speak and share.

The videos went viral.

I was inundated with hundreds of messages from people from all over the country saying they wished our services had been available when they lost their hair, or that they wished they were closer to us, or that they wanted to bring in their sister, their mother, a friend and most importantly, how amazing it was to see somebody who gets it. It was all confirmation that I was on the right track, that I was meant to be doing this.

What I came to realise after a few months was that some of the people coming in for wigs could afford to pay for them. But what about those who couldn't? Those were the ones who really needed our help. The people who had been through chemotherapy. The ones who couldn't work because of treatment. The ones whose futures had been thrown into uncertainty and whose incomes had been stripped from them.

My head was full once more with questions and annoyance. I needed to find a way to help all of these other women, and so I started to research again.

The next step was obvious: to become a supplier for the National Health Service, which meant I would have to bid for an NHS Procurement. It was every bit the nightmare it sounds. I went into researching the NHS Procurement bid process, spent months understanding the framework, contacted lots of different departments and searched for the right people to talk to.

This was challenging for somebody who had never written a tender, or a bid or even understood what the word "procurement" really meant.

I picked up the phone hundreds of times, not giving up but feeling like it was an impossible task. No one would answer - again and again. I'd be told there was nobody around to speak to. My emails went unanswered. It felt like an uphill struggle.

The life juggling was intense. I was trying to earn a living, manage my arthritis flares, run my hair salon, build a new business and to be honest, be able to say "no." I was exhausted and drained. But I kept going. My purpose was bigger and brighter. I was starting to realise that if I wanted to succeed in my mission, something had to change.

Bear in mind that I was still in recovery and my body was adapting to hormone therapy as I navigated chemically induced menopause at the age of 36. Amidst hot flushes, anxiety, and sleepless nights, I felt out of my depth, my brain was frazzled from being permanently switched on. The new habits that I was trying to implement sometimes fell by the wayside as I undertook this mammoth task of creating what I knew I was supposed to be doing.

I crashed emotionally and physically. I was petrified of being so run down that I invited the cancer back, so I had to give myself a talking-to: It was time to pause.

At the time, I was running on pure adrenaline, but I wouldn't and couldn't sacrifice my core business, time with my family or my health for everything and everybody else. It was a stark reminder that I was just as important as other people, and unless I was strong and healthy, I would be of no value to anyone.

It was time to ask for help. I wasn't sure how to do this, and it was a pretty uncomfortable thing for me - I was a strong, driven woman and loved pushing myself to achieve the next thing. I am proud of the fact that I could see I needed help because it was only with the right help that I'd move forward on my mission.

My salon up to this point was small and although financially stable and successful, I felt like I was just cutting hair and was certainly far from being a CEO. I saw myself as self-employed rather than running a business. This needed to change.

I did a few things: I joined a locally funded entrepreneur programme through Natwest Bank (thank you Nickie Killkenny and team) to broaden my skills and help me step into believing that I was a real entrepreneur, and I started to build a team. This was a total game-changer and was the best thing I did for myself and the business.

Three people came into my world who became angels for me personally and professionally. To this day, they are three of my most trusted and valuable team members. Alistair Nelson joined as my first new business employee, working one day a week - even that was a terrifying commitment. He came on board to help me get clear on the brand and our messaging. He's been instrumental in driving the business to where it is, working tirelessly over the years and is now running the operations as our COO.

The second person who started shifting things for me was Bev Mason. She'd come in to get her hair cut and we started chatting about what I was doing and how things were progressing. I just had this feeling – "I need you!" I was thinking to myself then. We still joke about how she came in for a haircut and left with a job. Having Bev take over as the office manager literally gave me so much value, including the thing I still treasure being able to do today, cutting my clients' hair and being the best part of their day or making them feel beautiful with or without hair.

Karen Young supported me to ensure I could recover and build the business I'd started dreaming about. Karen had been my mentor throughout my whole career and following her mum's recent cancer experience, was ready to jump in and help me. This was a stroke of luck for me and my wonderful clients to have Karen's expertise on board.

As you recover from cancer, it can be a relief to switch from worrying about your treatment and your cancer and all of the hospital stuff that goes with it to something new that you feel passionate about. Be careful that it does not take over. I didn't quite hit rock bottom, but I was close and heading there fast. Being able to recognise this and take control to make changes, was the pivotal moment the dial shifted in what I'd set out to build.

I will be forever grateful to the universe for aligning me with Alistair, Karen and Bev. And of course, those who further joined my team as we quickly gained momentum.

It worked, in November 2018, I received an email from Sunderland NHS Trust. I had successfully tendered for their wig contract. I burst into tears. This was my local hospital just a few minutes away from my salon. It was now possible to help people who simply could not afford a wig. Working alongside the NHS we could support all those people who were in that awful position of finding out they had cancer, likely going to lose their hair and probably had two or three weeks to get all their ducks in a row before it happened. These were the people who needed to be helped.

This is by far one of the proudest moments of my life. I could now help those who simply could not afford to buy a wig. I could work with the NHS and support all those people I'd seen as I sat and watched at the hospital.

Over the next five years, I actively managed and secured contracts with almost every hospital in the Northeast of England. I also earned a spot on the national NHS framework, enabling me to expand and franchise operations into other cities. I'm so proud that we have helped over 15,000 people with hair loss, and around 2,000 children and young people. It took a lot of work and I gradually built more skills and a small team to help me make it happen.

Then came Covid. Like the rest of the salons in the country, we were told to close our doors. We had seen it coming so had been frantically making videos of support and building supplies at home for stock we knew people still being diagnosed would need. Imagine dealing with cancer and the pandemic. A double sh*t show!

The country was in lockdown, and we had been ordered to close. We actively campaigned with our local MP to allow us to stay open. This was met with resistance. We told them, "No, we're not a salon, we are a healthcare provider. This is not cosmetic hairdressing; this is healthcare provision. We want to open and my team is willing. We need to be there for people." After much pushing and shoving, we got special permission and were allowed to stay open. Another triumph.

During Covid, I studied and became a trichologist to fully understand hair and scalp. This enabled me to speak to health professionals with knowledge and conviction, rather than just as a cancer patient or hairdresser. I began to speak at public events and offer keynotes and training courses to healthcare teams, teaching them about the true impact of hair loss on a person's well-being.

I proudly became an NHS volunteer and helped set up a team of community hairdressers who visited the local hospice to offer hair services – definitely my favourite day of the week. I took a role on the board of City and Guilds where I, as a trichologist, help steer the education of aspiring hairdressers to include more emphasis on hair loss.

My mission is simple: I want anyone experiencing hair loss to have access to a skilled, compassionate hair loss specialist, ideally in their own salon, a place where they already feel comfortable and understood. Every salon should have stylists who know how to handle both hair and hair loss with expertise and empathy. That's why we're partnering with salons across the country, ensuring they're trained not just in cutting and styling but also in the sensitive, life-changing support needed for clients facing hair loss. Hairdressers should know how to treat people with and without hair.

All of this is my way of giving something back and changing my narrative about cancer and its effects.

When I applied for and was selected to deliver a TED Talk – a short, impactful presentation where speakers share inspiring and thought-provoking ideas on various topics – I knew I was back and better than before. Standing on that red dot knowing how many people across the world could be positively impacted by those 12 minutes was absolutely terrifying. I wondered if my chest might burst onto all those sitting in the front row of the TED Talk auditorium; my heart was beating that fast. I spoke with integrity and purpose about the impact of hair loss.

Here I was standing on a red dot, my heart racing faster than a Saturday morning blow dry, speaking to thousands of people around the world about something that I felt so passionate about – the irony is not lost on me. Once a quivering wreck under the radiotherapy dots, now a nervous advocate on *the* red dot.

All because I had joined the Cancer Club.

My nana used to say, "God only gives you as much as you can handle," and I think that's relevant whether you believe in God or not. I have achieved all I have so far because of what I was given, cancer included. Believing that everything happens for a reason gives me hope, it gives me direction for the future and gets me out of bed every morning.

When you're in the thick of it, it can be difficult to see why it's happening to you, but as my story and the ones that follow will show you, there is always a reason, we just have to be willing to look.

21

Unbroken Strength

By Jo Knight

My story is that of a thousand women. I considered myself relatively healthy, a non-smoker and an occasional drinker, and I felt well. Breast cancer certainly wasn't part of my life plan, but it sneakily decided to take up residence behind my left breast.

In May 2017, at the age of 42, I received a diagnosis of Stage 2 breast cancer. I remember that day vividly when the bombshell dropped from a great height. The evil word that no one wants to hear. The fear and terror it instils, the uncertainty and unknown path that lies ahead. "Why me?" That is a question no one can answer.

After a whirlwind of tests and appointments, I started six sessions of chemotherapy, an experience I hope never to repeat. Knowing I'd lose my hair, I decided to take control. I shaved it all off. Cancer wasn't going to dictate how I felt about my appearance. Taking charge of how I looked was my way of telling myself that my identity wasn't tied to my hair or my looks.

Following chemotherapy, I was scheduled for surgery, and just before Christmas 2017, I had a bilateral mastectomy along with lymph node clearance on my left side. Oddly enough, this felt like the easiest part of the journey, I was finally getting rid of "Colin," the tumour that had invaded my body!

While many women struggle with the idea of losing their breasts, feeling as though it takes away from their femininity, I didn't have that same attachment.

By February 2018, I faced the final hurdle: 15 sessions of radiotherapy. I sailed through, with no major setbacks. By March, I was discharged from oncology. Elated? Yes. But it wasn't long before the reality hit me: no more hospital visits, just yearly check-ups and Tamoxifen. Alone with my thoughts, the mental weight of cancer set in.

Just as life was beginning to feel somewhat normal again, my periods came back with a vengeance. I decided to speak to my doctor, who referred me to a specialist. After numerous tests and examinations, and because my breast cancer was ER-positive, they recommended a full hysterectomy. In 2019, I underwent keyhole surgery to have it done.

I was lucky. My incredible family wrapped me in love and support. Without them and my warped sense of humour, this journey would have felt very different.

Be Bold, Be Brave, Be Beautiful, Be You

I'm nearly seven years post-cancer, and I still can't fully explain where my strength came from. Facing cancer, you dig deep. You pull on those big girl pants and march forward. It's been tough both physically and mentally. My scars are visible and hidden and they serve as daily reminders that although I'm cancer-free, it's never fully gone from my life.

Six years after treatment, I found out I have persistent chemotherapy-induced alopecia (PCIA). Only 3% of chemotherapy patients face long-term hair loss. My hair is patchy, thin and fluffy – and I'm not a fan. So, I embrace the shaved head and stylish scarves. My hair doesn't define me, neither do my boobs.

I turned to Instagram to share my journey. My goal? To help others navigate the same path. Raising awareness about regular checks and early detection is so important because it saves lives. I also advocate for "living flat" after mastectomies. Reconstruction isn't for everyone, and I want women to feel confident in their choices.

My body has transformed drastically over the past decade - JJ cups reduced to Ds and now, living flat. It's been a journey, but I believe women should feel proud and beautiful in their skin.

Preloved-Reloved Cancer and Beyond

Being a single mum and cancer survivor isn't easy. I've had a double mastectomy and a full hysterectomy, and I've dealt with hair loss that never fully recovered. Cancer brought some of the hardest moments in my life. Even with the love and support of my family, I often felt alone, scared and overwhelmed. But through those dark days, I found the strength to turn my pain into purpose.

That's when Preloved-Reloved Cancer and Beyond was born. My idea was simple: Provide free wigs, turbans, scarves, mastectomy pillows and clothing to those who need them. Not everyone can afford these essentials, and I wanted to make a difference.

I started a JustGiving page to cover postage costs, spread the word on Instagram and Facebook, and even visited hospitals and community spaces to reach people who needed help. And it worked.

Today, Preloved-Reloved is still a one-person operation, but the outpouring of support from the community has been incredible. Every story I hear from people I've helped drives me to keep going, to keep expanding this service. The messages of gratitude remind me that through my own struggle, I'm making a real difference. I'm determined to grow Preloved-Reloved to reach more regions, with drop-in centres and expanded services.

22

The Unseen Battle

by Suzanne Duncan

Cancer has taught me one critical lesson: Never take anything for granted. We often believe it won't happen to us, but it can. Cancer shifted my perspective, which allowed me to let go of trivial worries and focus on what truly matters.

The diagnosis was really blunt and a massive shock. I was reeling and in disbelief when I heard it. The pace at which things went after that was fast, with little time for processing. Despite the whirlwind, I tried to cling to my usual routine, stubbornly determined to maintain a sense of normality amidst the chaos.

Engaging in everyday activities became my anchor, a way to retain a semblance of control in the face of uncertainty. I made a conscious effort to keep my diagnosis as private as possible, seeking comfort in solitude as an introvert who hated gossip. Sharing the news meant surrendering a part of myself to the disease, as it often became the sole topic of conversation – something that I was reluctant to embrace. I carefully selected who to confide in, acutely aware that once the news was out, it couldn't be taken back. I felt that cancer not only challenged my physical health but also imposed a burden on my mental well-being, shaping how I navigated through my diagnosis and treatment journey.

People would share their fears and experiences of the disease, sometimes insensitively, for example sharing stories of their family members who had the disease and didn't survive. The more I heard these insensitive remarks, the more I desired to shield my mental health from further harm.

Physically, I found the treatment more manageable than I expected - once I got over my hospital phobia. But mentally, it was a fight. As a control freak, handing over my life to doctors was its own battle. My family, especially my husband and children, kept me going. My eldest said, "You're receiving treatment at the peak of medical science." His words were a reality check, such a wise child.

Overcoming Mental Strain

Losing my hair was one of the hardest parts. I was determined to keep the diagnosis private, but hair loss threatened that. It wasn't just about the change in appearance. Hair had been a significant part of my identity. I hadn't realised how much I valued it until it was gone.

Losing my fingernails at the end of treatment was another blow. It surprised me how much I missed them and how I had overlooked their importance. Unlike my toenails, which are easier to conceal, losing my fingernails was a visible reminder of my body's struggles.

While hair loss is a well-known side effect of treatment, nail loss caught me off guard and added to my feelings of falling apart. I was grateful that my nails grew back much quicker than my hair.

I discovered the importance of nurturing my mental well-being alongside my physical health. Cancer challenges the mind as much as the body, and I found solace in simple pleasures like treating myself to a facial, enjoying a coffee with a friend, diving into a good book and even planning future holidays.

These activities became my coping mechanisms, providing moments of joy whilst simultaneously going through the turmoil of treatment.

Setting goals, whether it was completing a book or planning a getaway, gave me a sense of purpose and direction during a time when everything else felt uncertain.

One of my greatest discoveries was a wig specialist, almost by accident. It sounds silly, but finding the perfect wig was a lifesaver. The compassion and care I received made me feel like myself again. It was a reminder that I could get through this, and it gave me the confidence to face the world.

Sometimes, I found myself liking the new hair more than the old. The compliments boosted my self-esteem, and I appreciated the knowledge I gained about wig care. Who knew hair not attached to your head could have its perks? Maintaining my newfound "hair armour" left me feeling empowered once again.

A New Perspective

Cancer is as much a battle of the mind as it is of the body. I had to stop overthinking and take each day as it came. Instead of drowning myself in online forums, I started connecting with people who had gone through similar journeys. Sharing my story was hard but also healing. It reminded me how far I'd come and, more importantly, that I could help someone else navigate their path.

I made myself a playlist for treatment – songs like "Staying Alive" by the Bee Gees never failed to lift my mood. It sounds trivial, but these little joys became crucial in keeping my spirits up.

Cancer forced me to redefine how I lived, and in many ways, it made me stronger. Not just in the body but in the mind too.

23

Learning Not to Take It Personally

By May Dargue

I first learned about my leukaemia diagnosis on what was supposed to be one of the best days of my life – my last day of school. I was getting ready to celebrate when the call came. The doctors asked me to come in immediately, and I was in complete shock. It didn't even occur to me how serious this was. I even asked if I could take my final exam first. But when I got to the doctor's, I was told I had to go straight to the Royal Victoria Infirmary. I had been referred there as an emergency.

Everything happened so fast, and it was impossible to grasp the enormity of the situation. My life had suddenly been turned upside down, and all my plans for the summer and sixth form disappeared. I felt completely lost.

The chemotherapy was intense. I had four rounds between June and December, and it hit me hard. Losing my independence was one of the hardest things to come to terms with, but the worst part was losing my hair. My hair has always been a huge part of my identity. It was what people noticed about me first. After it fell out, I didn't recognise myself anymore.

Accepting help from others was difficult, too. I had to rely on people for even the smallest tasks. The chemo also killed my appetite, and I lost a lot of weight. This made me physically weaker and impacted my entire routine. But my diagnosis also showed me who was truly there for me, and it made me stronger and more resilient in the long run.

Before the illness, my life had been so social - school, a job, going out with friends. I had to watch from the sidelines as everyone attended prom and enjoyed summer plans, I was supposed to be part of. It was heartbreaking in a way that only those who've gone through chemotherapy can truly understand.

Beyond the Diagnosis

Throughout the hardest moments, my mam was my rock. She gave me space to process my emotions and always listened without judgement. Her presence made me feel safe, and I couldn't have managed without her. The nurses were also incredible; they treated me like a person, not just a patient, which made all the difference.

Social media became too painful to look at, so I stayed off it. Seeing my friends live out the life I felt cut off from made it harder to cope. At night, when sleep was hard to come by, I found solace in focusing on my breathing to calm myself down.

Writing helped too. Whenever I was overwhelmed, I'd jot down my thoughts and feelings. It was a way to release emotions when I wasn't ready to talk. Over time, it became a way to track how much I had grown and overcome.

My friends, Emma and Amy, also played a big role in getting me through it all. They helped me vent, and their support reminded me that I wasn't alone. They normalised my feelings and reassured me when I needed it most.

Rediscovering Myself Through Wigs

When I started wearing wigs, it was awkward at first. I was so self-conscious, worried that people would stare, but in reality, the wig looked completely natural. Eventually, it gave me back my confidence. I started to feel pretty again. I was no longer just the girl who had lost her hair - I was someone with a new identity, a fresh start. This "new me" wasn't just about the wig or makeup, it was about regaining control of how I presented myself to the world.

Playing around with different wigs became a fun way to experiment with my appearance. I even dyed one wig red, a colour I never would have tried with my natural hair. It was like stepping into a new role each day. Turning it into a positive experience, rather than dwelling on what I had lost, gave me strength.

The Emotional Toll of Words

People don't always know what to say, and I learned quickly not to take their comments personally. Some friends complained about having to go to work or college, not realising how much I longed for that normality. One friend even mentioned being jealous of my hair before the illness - an innocent comment, but it stung deeply because I still hadn't fully accepted the loss.

My advice to anyone supporting a loved one through chemotherapy? Be patient and understanding. If they lash out, know it's the pain talking. And for those going through it - don't be afraid to ask for help. It's okay to talk to someone and admit that you're struggling. There's strength in seeking support.

Finding My Strength and Moving Forward

Cancer taught me not to look too far into the future – it's overwhelming. Instead, I learned to take things day by day. I discovered I'm stronger than I ever imagined, both physically and mentally. For anyone else going through it, be kind to yourself. You're not just a cancer patient; you're a person navigating life's toughest challenges. Take pride in how far you've come.

Now that I'm healthy, I'm eager to live life to the fullest. After spending half a year in the hospital, I'm making up for lost time with friends and family. I've planned trips, concerts and days out. But most importantly, I've surrounded myself with people who love and support me. It's made all the difference in starting to socialise again after such a daunting journey.

Going back to work was a huge milestone. It gave me a sense of purpose and a reason to get out of bed each day. I'm so grateful to be here, healthy and ready to embrace life. Cancer has given me a mindset of gratitude and resilience. It's shown me that even after the hardest battles, there's always room for joy.

24

Words That Heal

Anonymous

I'll share my story from three different perspectives: as a child with a parent battling cancer, as a friend of someone dear facing cancer, and as a healthcare professional with 35 years of experience in cancer and palliative care.

Reflections on My Dad's Cancer Journey

In 1983, when I was just 12, my carefree world turned upside down. My father, only 42 at the time, was diagnosed with a rare blood disorder called angioimmunoblastic lymphadenopathy. The medical jargon was beyond my comprehension, and significantly, the word "cancer" was never spoken. The absence of that single word both shielded and confused us. My father's health deteriorated rapidly, his energy drained, his hair fell out and he grew irritable. My siblings and I carried on with our lives, oblivious to the gravity of his condition, while my mother and grandmother quietly supported him through his treatments.

In hindsight, the choice to avoid using the word "cancer" may have been an attempt to protect us, but it also kept us in the dark. Without understanding the full reality of what was happening, we were left unprepared for the emotional toll. Looking back, I realise how vital honest, clear communication could have been for my family. It would have allowed us to better understand his illness, and given us the tools to cope with it.

After eight months, his treatments stopped, and slowly but surely, my father's strength returned. It felt like we could breathe again, and life returned to normal. But a decade later, when a lump appeared under his arm, the truth became undeniable - he had cancer. This time, there was no shielding us. As a qualified nurse specialising in haematology by then, I felt the weight of the diagnosis deeply. I was no longer just his daughter; I became his caregiver. I had the privilege of ensuring he received the best possible care during his final years until his passing in 1995.

His journey taught me the importance of transparency in these difficult conversations. The absence of resources at the time was frustrating, but I'm thankful for organisations like Macmillan that now provide the emotional and practical support we could have used back then.

A Friend's Perspective

In 2018, my best friend, my rock through life's challenges, was diagnosed with breast cancer. I'll never forget the shock I felt. This woman, my pillar of strength, now faced her own storm. Despite it feeling so unfair, I knew it was my turn to stand by her.

Her approach to the diagnosis was pragmatic, almost stoic. "What will be, will be," she would often say. As a nurse with experience in cancer services, she knew more than most, sometimes that knowledge was helpful, and sometimes it weighed heavily on her. She had a clear plan: "One shot at everything - no second chances, no clinical trials." Her decision was final. Reflecting on her journey, I've come to understand the power of language.

Her family, understandably, was devastated by the news. That's when "Philomena" entered the scene - a little worry monster we made together. We'd write down our fears, and feed them to Philomena, and somehow, it lightened the load. Six years on, Philomena still sits in her living room, a reminder that laughter and comfort can exist in the darkest times.

Chemotherapy was especially tough for her. As we prepared for her hair loss, she made the brave decision to shave it all off ahead of time. Our trips to the hairdresser became ritualistic, and I was in awe of her strength. Fortunately, we have a fabulous hairdresser - the one who has written this book! We even found a fantastic wig that matched her natural hair, helping her maintain a semblance of normalcy during her treatment. Beneath her brave demeanour, I could sense that it was a tough time for her.

Her treatment plan involved surgery followed by six cycles of chemotherapy and then radiotherapy, which was undoubtedly a tough road. Surgery proceeded smoothly, allowing for a few weeks of recovery before beginning chemotherapy. But the chemotherapy wreaked havoc on her veins, eventually leading to complications. After four cycles, she fell seriously ill and was hospitalised with what we suspect was sepsis. Faced with a choice, she decided to stop chemotherapy, choosing quality of life over continuing treatment.

Even as she fought cancer, she did so with grace and determination. The next stage was radiotherapy, which she faced with the same resolve. Today, she's cancer-free, and her resilience continues to inspire me.

What I've learned as a Nurse and Supporter

With 35 years in cancer and palliative care, I've learned some invaluable lessons. If I could sum it up, it's this: Don't give unsolicited advice. Everyone's journey is their own, and you can never fully understand how you would react until you're in that situation. Sometimes, the best thing you can offer is your presence, not your words.

The words we choose can either uplift or burden those we love. Too often, we rush to fill silence with our thoughts, but silence can be comforting too. There's no universal script for supporting someone through cancer, but I've seen time and again that small gestures, whether it's a listening ear, a shared cup of tea, or just sitting quietly beside someone – can mean more than we realise.

If you're going through cancer, know this: You are unique, and so is your journey. Don't let anyone dictate how you should feel or act. Lean on those who understand, be honest about your needs, and give yourself permission to feel what you're feeling. You are in charge of your story.

Cancer is just a word - it carries many meanings and many outcomes, but it doesn't define you. You define your journey. And remember, sometimes the smallest acts of kindness or understanding can make the biggest difference.

25

Resilience from Childhood

By Kat Watson-Wood

At the age of four, just two days after my birthday, my life was thrown off course when I was diagnosed with a tangerine-sized tumour on the cerebellum of my brain, the part responsible for balance. The news shook my family, setting off a whirlwind of treatments. I underwent both radiotherapy and surgery to combat the disease, and to this day, I continue to be monitored by Christie's due to the long-term effects of radiation on my pituitary gland. Only now, at 36, do I truly appreciate the magnitude of what I went through and how fortunate I am to still be here.

While I don't remember much about the surgery itself, certain moments stick out in my memory. The smell of hospital corridors, the bumpy ride on the theatre trolley, and the nurse who hastily ripped off my ECG sticker, which my mum later joked about, calling it my "third nipple," when I went for radiotherapy, the plaster of Paris helmet, the "tissue box" that I had to put my face in and the excruciating pain when the nurse removed the stitches from my "zip" wound down the back of my neck.

There are also more comforting memories, like the blackcurrant cordial I was given and the spaghetti on toast I ate when I arrived at the hospital. These small, vivid memories are what remain with me from that tumultuous time.

Throughout everything, my parents were my unwavering support. They still are to this day. Even as an adult, they accompany me to appointments, stepping in to advocate for me when I can't, treating me like any other "normal" child. They always encouraged me to try new things, even when my body sometimes couldn't keep up with other children.

Growing up, I had to mature quickly due to my health, but I wasn't short on academic help. Coming from a family of teachers, I was well-supported with schoolwork, even as I struggled with undiagnosed dyslexia. However, with everything going on, I didn't have many friends, and my health challenges made fitting in a bit more difficult. It wasn't until the pandemic that I started to fully grasp the enormity of my journey, and I felt compelled to start sharing my story to help others who might be facing something similar.

From an early age, I wanted to help people just as the nurses and therapy staff had helped me. Little did I know that pursuing a career in nursing would be so physically challenging due to my limb weakness, balance issues and fatigue. Despite these obstacles, I worked incredibly hard at school and graduated from university in 2009 with a degree in adult nursing studies.

Where the Cancer Journey Led Me

After 15 years of working in care homes and on hospital wards, it became clear that the long-term effects of my cancer treatments were making it too difficult to continue such physically demanding work. My body was telling me it was time for a change. I shifted into a role as a Disability Advisor, helping people with different conditions get the support they needed. This transition felt like a natural extension of my nursing career. A deaf patient I worked with even inspired me to learn sign language, allowing me to conduct consultations in British Sign Language (BSL) and make a real difference in their care.

But as the effects of radiation continued to take their toll, I realised it was time to step back and look after myself. After years of taking care of others, I needed to prioritise my health. Reflecting on my journey over the past 30 years, I feel incredibly proud of everything I've accomplished, and I now want to share my experiences with others to give them hope and support. It's important to know that you're not alone.

Currently, I work for an IT sales company and have become a founding member of their disability and neurodiversity network. My nursing background continues to influence my work as I provide support and advice to others, using both my professional experience and personal journey.

Be ready to open up about your experiences. Don't hesitate to share your story, as it can be empowering and inspiring, especially for those facing similar challenges. Remember, you're stronger than whatever challenges you're facing. Cancer inspired me to help others, leading me to work with our disability network at my workplace, where I offer support and advice on coping strategies and reasonable adjustments.

Often, when faced with negativity, I find solace in humour, choosing to laugh at myself – a coping mechanism many of us with neurodiverse conditions use. My blue badge is affectionately referred to as my "biddy badge" by my friends – my bestie tells me the only reason I have friends is because I get cheap theatre tickets and the best parking spaces!

The support I've received from The Christie Hospital in Manchester since 1992 has been a lifeline, and I now participate in brain tumour research and charity events to raise awareness about cancer survivorship.

I firmly believe that with the right mindset, anything is possible. Having worked as a nurse for 15 years, I've seen firsthand how a positive outlook can transform a situation. It's essential to use your experiences, whether good or bad, to help others facing similar journeys. Sharing your story can be incredibly empowering, and I hope mine inspires others to realise their strength.

26

A Mother's Legacy

By Nikki Hall

Many people have told me "You are so strong." But I know that challenges in life are relative. For someone with a solid support system and no financial worries, what might seem like a massive challenge can feel easier to face than what appears as a small challenge to someone battling alone. Through experience, I've learned that the principles of facing adversity remain the same, no matter the circumstances.

When I was 12, my mum passed away from breast cancer at just 38. This event marked my life in a way I couldn't fully grasp at the time. As a result of her passing, I was placed on a cancer screening program, going for yearly checks. At the time, I didn't think much of it, it became part of my routine. If it weren't for my mum's death, I would never have been so diligent about screening. In many ways, my mum's loss saved my life.

At age 45, during my annual check-up, I was diagnosed with Grade 1 breast cancer. The shock of it didn't hit me all at once, but soon, I found myself in a whirlwind of appointments and decisions. I had one mastectomy and, although I wasn't a carrier of the BRCA gene, I chose to undergo a second mastectomy as a preventative measure.

The diagnosis was life-changing in ways I hadn't anticipated. I remember someone telling me, "You can instantly write off a year of your life when you're diagnosed with cancer," and they were right. My wedding plans had to be put on hold as recovery took both physical and emotional tolls. While people celebrate when you are declared cancer-free, the journey for the patient is far from over. It's just the beginning of a new chapter.

I was incredibly fortunate to have a loving husband who supported me through every surgery, offering the practical help I needed to recover. My son and my close friends were equally invaluable, ensuring I stayed open about my feelings. Losing both breasts and confronting the scars was challenging.

To this day, I remind myself that these scars are proof that my life was saved. Small acts of kindness from a friend's comforting words to an unexpected card, pulled me through in ways I'll never forget.

One realisation hit me harder than anything else: My mum's death saved my life. Without her, I wouldn't have been on the screening program. By the time I would have noticed a lump, it might have been too late. That understanding stayed with me, and I felt a deep sense of gratitude mixed with sorrow.

My mum's legacy wasn't just her love but the lifesaving practice of early detection. Once I recovered, I knew I had a mission: to raise awareness about the importance of screenings and regular checks. I wanted to help save other lives the way mine had been saved.

One Step at a Time

One of the ways I chose to honour that mission was by taking on a huge challenge: climbing Mount Kilimanjaro. A year after my final surgery, I set out to conquer the mountain, not only to raise awareness but also to raise funds for a local cancer charity that had supported me during treatment. The generosity of people amazed me, and the climb became one of the most significant experiences of my life. I'm still in touch with the five women I met through the charity, and their support continues to mean the world to me.

Reaching the summit of Kilimanjaro on 19 September 2019 was a personal victory, both physically and mentally. The "one step at a time" approach I had applied to cancer treatment helped me take on this mountain, too. There were moments of vulnerability, but that's what made it so empowering.

Being surrounded by strangers on that climb, I felt a strong sense of connection. It reminded me that you don't have to know someone well to feel supported. The shared experience was enough. Climbing that mountain was about reclaiming my confidence and proving to myself that I could face the toughest challenges head-on.

Through social media, radio interviews and word of mouth, I've been able to share my story in the hope of encouraging others to prioritise their health. Connecting with people, whether over a cup of coffee or through a quick message, has made this journey so much richer. My story isn't just about survival but about being proactive.

I've always believed that small, everyday actions can save lives. Screenings, self-checks or even just talking about it, those things matter. By posting regularly about my own experiences, I hoped to encourage others to take their health seriously and not to ignore any warning signs.

A Legacy of Laughter and Love

Breast cancer is something I would never wish on anyone, but it has brought unexpected blessings into my life, too. I've found humour to be a great ally through it all. My surgeon, for example, would sketch all over my chest like a puzzle, figuring out the best way to save my nipples while removing the breasts – a bit like playing dot-to-dot. My husband, an engineer, watched in fascination, while I couldn't help but laugh.

I've learned that much of the stress in these situations comes from the mind. Staying positive, focusing on small victories and taking things one step at a time has been key to getting through. Cancer has also made me more empathetic and I know that we never truly understand someone's struggles. Just because they've survived doesn't mean they aren't still carrying invisible scars.

For all the challenges cancer brought, it has also brought many wonderful things into my life: deep connections, laughter, and a renewed appreciation for every moment. My mum's legacy continues to shape me, and through my journey, I hope to help others find strength in their own stories.

27

The Beauty in Surrender

By Arjuna Ishaya

Both of my mums died from cancer. My real mum was initially diagnosed with cancer in her brain, lungs and liver. She underwent treatment, but, looking back, she didn't stand a chance.

I flew back to New Zealand from the UK and waited. For a disease with such an aggressive reputation, cancer can be mind-numbingly slow. I found myself making cups of coffee, mowing the lawn, driving her to appointments and handing her the TV remote when she mistakenly tried to change channels with her phone. I'd jump into action to make whatever food she might be able to taste, given the damage chemotherapy had done to her taste buds.

Gone were my visions of riding in on a white horse, introducing her to all my friends in the alternative health space, and watching her make a miraculous recovery. I imagined her doctors standing in awe while I sat in the background, smiling smugly. But that was my plan, she had her own. She was making her own choices. I could either fight and insist or I could surrender to her will.

There's an old saying: "Do you want to be right, or do you want to be happy?" It seems simple when framed that way, doesn't it? I chose to support her, with no demands attached. I decided to be of service, to enjoy whatever time we had together, rather than insisting that my way was best for her.

At that moment, I didn't have a plan for my own life. It was all about her. When I let my guard down, I resented her. I wished she would hurry up and die so I could get on with my own life. Caregivers will understand that feeling. Then, guilt would wash over me, and I'd use it as a reminder to adjust my attitude. I chose to be there; I wanted to be there. It was up to me to make the most of the moments I had with her, my family and life itself.

I had to be careful in my mind. It was so easy to slip into the darkness of past regrets or future fears. I'd catch myself spiralling – imagining mum getting worse, the doctors saying it was over and seeing myself sobbing at her funeral. But then, I'd snap back to the present. There she was, asking for another cup of tea or talking about her roses. Those "What if" daydreams stole time and gave nothing in return but suffering.

That was one of the sharpest and most beautiful lessons I learned: suffering became the alarm bell, reminding me to cherish what was most precious. I couldn't afford to dilly-dally in the dark corners of my mind. Life was happening now – Mum was here now.

In truth, I didn't "do" much. But just before she died, Mum thanked me. She said I was the only one who wasn't rushing around in a tizzy, the only one who didn't seem to want anything from her. I wasn't afraid of what life would look like without her. All I did was sit and be present, and that turned out to be enough to make her final days a little better.

Losing my mum strengthened my bond with my brother. We weren't close before, but we had time to sit together, talk and apologise for the past. In some ways, I'm grateful for that.

Life has a way of balancing things out. People leave, but others come into your life. I saw this most clearly when I got a call about an old girlfriend who had taken her own life. Moments later, my brother called to announce the birth of his son.

There's always a why in life. But scratching at that scab doesn't bring answers, it just leaves scars. You have to find a way to accept the why and put it to rest. Sometimes, all you can do is shrug and say, "It is what it is." Let it be until it starts to make sense on its own. Patience is a fine thing.

A psychologist once talked about skilled versus unskilled attitudes and actions. The lesson I've learned is that life gives you what it gives you, and you can either handle it skillfully or not. It doesn't have to weigh so heavily. Grieving, yes, but even grief can be light. As they say, "Pain is inevitable, but suffering is optional."

This is one of the lessons of all of this. This is part of the "Why?" we seek. We make it. We choose. We get to define. What we focus on, grows. We get to decide how we live and die, and the great thing is that no one or nothing can take that away from us.

My mother-in-law also had her own dance with cancer, lasting sixteen years. She lost both breasts, her hair fell out three times, and her arm swelled monstrously after lymph nodes were removed. My wife had to alter her clothing to fit the swelling. But the word "battle" doesn't suit her story.

She embodied grace. There was no fight in her. Rather than focusing on destroying cancer, she focused on what was beautiful and good. She patted her shoulder regularly, saying, "Well done, body, you're doing the very best you can." I even tried it when I had a cold, and found gratitude to be a powerful foundation for healing. It made everything feel lighter, easier and more expansive because I was focusing on what I had, not what I lacked.

Her journey was about peace. Not waiting for things to change, but accepting them as they were and living fully in that moment. At the end of her life, she was small and shrunken, but her eyes were huge and bright. In one of her moments of clarity, she looked at me, full of joy, and said, "I get to find out what happens next!"

I know she had doubts and fears, but she was inspirational in consciously and consistently returning to gratitude and appreciation and not taking anything for granted - and in that, she showed me how to live with style.

Be open. Pay attention. Stay curious. Get inquisitive. Focus on what you can do, not what you can't. Stay with what you've got, not what you have not. Take what you're given and create as much good from it as you can.

Anthony de Mello, author and psychotherapist, was once asked about life after death. He said, "'Life after death?' Is there life before death? That is the question!"

28

Reflections from Specialist Cancer Nurses

By Michele Hughes and Sue Longstaff

Editor's note: Michele Hughes is a Clinical Nurse Specialist for Oncology and Sue Longstaff is a Lung Cancer Nurse Specialist. What follows is a list of reminders and reflections from two professionals.

We've both spent years working with cancer patients, and over time, certain things become clearer. There are lessons, reminders, and a bit of advice we've gathered, some from our experiences, others from the people we've met along the way. If you or someone close to you is on a cancer journey, here are some thoughts we'd like to share:

First off, chemo doesn't affect everyone the same way. Some people get sick, others don't. Just because someone had a terrible reaction doesn't mean you will too. We're all unique, and cancer treatment doesn't follow a single path for everyone. Keep us informed. If something doesn't feel right or if side effects are creeping in, tell us. We can help, but only if we know. Trust your body, and trust that you have a team behind you ready to adjust, assist and support.

One of the biggest misconceptions we see is that people assume they should just "get through" the tough times on their own. Please don't isolate yourself. If you feel like you can't face the day or if getting out of bed seems impossible, take a breath. Ask yourself if it's a physical barrier or emotional exhaustion and then reach out. We've been through these moments with many patients, and there's always a way forward.

There's no such thing as a silly question. If something is bothering you, whether it's a physical symptom or an anxious thought, speak up. We'd rather answer 100 questions than let one unasked question lead to unnecessary worry.

Here's a gentle reminder: Dr. Google isn't always your friend. It's tempting to search for every side effect or symptom, but this often leads to more anxiety than answers. The internet is full of conflicting information. Focus on what your doctors and nurses are telling you and lean on them for clarity. We're here to guide you through this maze.

For those dealing with breast cancer, understand that it's not just one type of cancer. There are many forms, and each one has its treatment plan.

That's why you could be in a room full of people with breast cancer and notice everyone is getting different drugs or schedules. It's normal and it's tailored to you.

One of the hardest parts of the journey is hair loss. It can change the way you see yourself. It's not just about losing hair; it's about seeing a different face in the mirror every day.

We get it. Know that for most people, it's temporary, and while that doesn't take away the difficulty, it might provide some light at the end of the tunnel. You're still you, no matter how different the reflection may seem.

Parents, if your child has been diagnosed with cancer, it's important to coordinate with family, friends, and even teachers about how to talk about it. Consistency in language and approach can help kids feel more secure.

Don't be afraid to show emotions around your children. It's okay to let them see you're sad or unwell some days. Kids take their emotional cues from you. If you pull away or shut down, they might do the same. Be open and let them know it's safe to feel what they're feeling.

Exercise can be a great ally during treatment. We're not talking about hitting the gym hard, but gentle movement can help lift your spirits and keep your body more resilient. Find what feels right for you, but don't push your body too hard. A balanced, healthy diet and hydration are just as crucial, no need for radical diets or fitness regimes. Keep it simple, listen to your body, and nourish it well.

For partners, intimacy and touch remain important parts of a relationship. Even when it feels like everything is changing, small gestures: a hug, or holding hands, are powerful reminders that love and connection remain constant. If side effects creep up or something feels off, don't try to figure it out on your own. Call the helpline. That's what it's there for so you don't have to guess, worry, or make decisions in isolation. The sooner you reach out, the better we can help.

And lastly, be kind to yourself. There will be bad days, and it's okay to feel low or angry. Staying positive all the time is exhausting. Take breaks, ask for help, and talk to someone you trust. Being honest with family and friends allows them to be there for you in ways you might not expect.

Sometimes, it's the smallest things - talking, resting and letting someone else handle the cooking - that makes the biggest difference. You're not alone in this, and with honesty, patience and openness, you'll find the support you need to carry you through.

Reflections from Nicola

Turns out, losing your hair and living your life without boobs can't stop you from living life to the fullest.

Cancer challenges the mind as much as the body and maintaining normality and privacy can be essential coping strategies, even when battling mental and physical tolls.

Learning how to detach from others' comments, as May did, and investing in personal growth enables you to reclaim a sense of self after diagnosis.

Cancer may be hard to explain, but honestly, if you can get through talking about it, you can handle just about anything - even when Philomena the worry monster eats your concerns for breakfast!

Surviving childhood cancer shaped Kat's perspective on life, inspiring her career as a nurse and ongoing advocacy, proving that even life's hardest challenges can lead to helping others.

Nikki reflects on how her mother's death ultimately saved her life, reinforcing the importance of regular screenings and how personal tragedy can inspire individuals to support others facing similar circumstances.

It turns out that sometimes being the best caregiver means mastering the art of making tea, hunting for TV remotes and accepting that life's greatest gift is simply showing up.

Practical advice from oncology nurses reminds us that communication, self-care, and understanding one's individual cancer journey are critical in navigating the challenges of treatment and recovery.

Chapter 5
Rising from the Shadows

So much has changed in the years since my diagnosis. None of it I could have imagined when the doctor first told me I had breast cancer. Out of all the possibilities and situations, the potential futures, and even the lack of one, that I saw in that moment, this was not one of them – and therefore, I am incredibly grateful for how my story has unfolded.

At the beginning of my journey, you wouldn't have been able to tell I was going through cancer. My industry was all about hair, beauty and confidence – you might catch me in a tracksuit with no makeup at home, but when I leave the house, I'm the type to paint my face and dress at least half decently. It was always how I dealt with the big things in life. I try to look my absolute best for big meetings or events, meeting new people and the like. If I look good, then everything will go well.

I call this my "tits and teeth" expression. Pull your shoulders back, stand tall, push out your chest, and flash that smile. My friend Sabine calls it the Peggy Mitchell face, the character from *Eastenders*. It's the way she'd be screaming and shouting in her home at the back of the bar and then come walking through the curtain with a huge smile and a "What can I get ya, darlin'?" My "tits and teeth" strategy has never failed me.

Approaching my cancer appointments with this strategy gave me a certain level of control. I would be ridiculously overdressed for every single one. My doctors and nurses thought it was hilarious. They'd ask where I was headed, and I'd cheekily reply "Well, I'm coming here." In my head, I'd be thinking that nobody could give me bad news if I looked and felt great.

On the day of my surgery, I couldn't bring anything into the operating room. I lay there waiting with no makeup on, no blow dry, no nails - just me. It was so quiet in that room, until my doctor, a big jolly man, came bounding in through the double doors and started bellowing with laughter. He reached into his pocket to bring out his phone. "What in the world are you doing?" I asked him. "This is the first time I have ever seen you without makeup, and I'm going to take your picture so I can blackmail you with it for the rest of your life," he told me. We burst into laughter.

That day was the first and last time my doctor ever saw me without makeup, but more importantly, that was the day he saved my life. That surgery was the start of a long journey towards healing, both literally and figuratively. It would take me years to be comfortable again in my own body, as my new self. Us laughing together in the operating room was one of the few moments I'd had in a very long time where I was just a human connecting with another human.

Before my radiotherapy part of the treatment commenced, I had to go and have some tattoos put on my body so that the radiation would hit exactly the right spot. It was utterly fascinating, but I also felt dehumanised. I think this was the most upset I became throughout all of my treatment.

I lay on a bed that reminded me of Aslan's deathbed in *The Lion, The Witch and the Wardrobe*. I had been measured millimetre-perfect and lined up with lasers across the ceilings. I had tiny little dots of tattoos marked across my chest with a pinprick. It wasn't painful, it was scary and surreal. I got so upset afterwards and cried for hours - I couldn't stop the tears. Every time I looked down, I saw these little tattoos, tiny dots, reminders that I was not out of the woods yet. These dots would save my heart from being radiated within an inch of its life. They reminded me that this was serious shit.

Every once in a while, during my treatment period, I would let myself enjoy bits of normality, usually with help from the medical professionals treating me. Caroline, my nurse at the Queen Elizabeth, was my guiding light. She explained everything so well and never let me feel stupid for asking questions.

There was also the cracking young Irish man who took care of me during my radiotherapy sessions. Whenever I went in, he would be ready with headphones and music.

On my initial visit, he asked me what I wanted to listen to and I replied, "Old-school hip-hop," which he found amusing. He explained that he's usually asked for Rod Stewart, Elton John and The Eagles. "No one's asked for Dr. Dre before!" My Irish radiographer would welcome me with a new playlist of banging tunes each day - the only downside to this was having to stay super still and not be able to jump on the bed and shake my booty! These humble and incredible people all helped me through my treatment.

It may sound morbid, but as any cancer survivor will tell you, a happy ending is not our default belief. There were times when I could not allow myself to believe in a positive outcome. The human brain has an average of 9:1 negative thought bias. Throw cancer in the mix and you can see why it's hard some days to be "tits and teeth"!

It took deep digging from within, drawing from my strength. Random connections with others, strong relationships with friends and family, and a purpose; all came together to help me feel glimmers of hope. I didn't wake up one day and suddenly believe that I'd make it all the way through, like sunshine and birds breaking through the horizon, but I found little things that I could hold on to and started to build on those.

Cancer changes everything. It took its toll on me in all the ways it could. It changed my perspective on what it means to really *live*. Cancer gave me a chance to step off the hamster wheel of life. The constant pressure to be Superwoman, to please everyone, to excel in every role - mam, wife, businesswoman - disappeared. With each year that passed, I took time to stop, reflect and re-evaluate what it was I truly wanted and allowed myself space to change.

I appreciated the value of life and no longer wanted to keep working to the point of breakdown. I reframed my priorities and looked upon my business and mission as a gift. I'm still having to make sure I pause and tweak my lifestyle so I am living the way I want to and I love that I get to do this because of cancer. If I'd not had cancer and slowed that hamster wheel right down, I would have simply kept it spinning and never stopped.

The upcoming stories in this chapter all revolve around a common theme: incredible individuals allowing themselves to embrace certain feelings and actions. Allowing yourself to hope is arguably the biggest gamble you could take in any context, but when we're talking about cancer, the stakes are so much higher – but so are the rewards. I was cautious about it, but I did allow myself to hope. I gathered the glimmers of hope over the years, and because I believed, I dared to work towards a future, one I am still fighting for.

It doesn't always have to be grand. These stories highlight the importance of acknowledging and accepting small moments of happiness too, whether it's enjoying a warm cup of tea or sharing a tender moment with loved ones. It is often these simple things that lead to hope and building courage.

29

The Courage to Feel

By Ashleigh Palmer

My view of life has completely transformed, and I've learned to find joy in the small, everyday moments. But I am aware that life can change in an instant. One day, while applying moisturiser, I discovered a lump on my collarbone. Everyone around me reassured me it was nothing - just a pulled muscle from the gym. But I couldn't shake the feeling that something wasn't right.

It took a month of ignoring my gut before I finally booked a GP appointment, squeezing it into my hectic schedule with the kids in tow. The doctor wasn't alarmed, but I couldn't let go of the unease. A hospital visit soon followed, kids still tagging along.

And then came that look. The one from the technician during the ultrasound that sent my heart into overdrive. When the follow-up call came, my worst fear was realised. Cancer. My world spun out of control as I collapsed into my parents' arms, sobbing.

"Cancer? At my age?" I thought. "How could this be happening to me? A young, fit mother of three little ones, ages seven, three, and two?" The emotions came in waves – fear, disbelief and anger all tangled together. It felt like life was happening to someone else.

But early in my journey, I made a crucial decision. I would allow myself to feel everything, to experience every emotion. Suppressing those feelings would have only added unnecessary stress. I knew I had to face them head-on, even if that meant sitting with the sadness, the anger and the fear. Days became a blur of tests, scans and meetings with specialists. And then came the diagnosis, Stage 2 Hodgkin's Lymphoma. With it came a six-month marathon of intense chemotherapy. As a mum, my biggest concern was my kids. How would I care for them? How could I make sure they were okay? I began writing letters to them, pouring my heart out, hoping to leave something behind for them if the worst happened.

Nights were often the hardest. In those dark hours, I clung to my husband, both of us terrified of what the future might bring. Yet, through those raw, emotional moments, we found a deeper connection. The honesty of sharing our fears brought us closer than ever before.

Even in the middle of it all, I found glimmers of hope. I decided to donate my hair to the Little Princess Trust, and it felt like I was turning my hardship into something meaningful. That decision gave me a sense of purpose. But with chemotherapy came inevitable hair loss, and by the second round, it was falling out rapidly. The moment I realised I had to shave my head was hard, but thanks to Nicola from The Wonderful Wig Company, it didn't feel as devastating as I thought. She helped me find a wig that looked just like my natural hair, something that felt like "me."

But no matter how hard you try to stay positive, some days hit like a freight train. By my 10th round of chemo, I was struggling. There were days when I didn't want to leave the house, let alone go on a school trip with my kids. And just when I thought I'd finished the worst of it, eight months after my final treatment, I relapsed. It felt like everything had been for nothing. Back to square one, with more chemo and a stem cell transplant on the horizon.

The relapse shook me. My family, including my husband, my mam and my dad, were all on edge. We had emotional, tear-filled arguments. Everyone was scared.

But then, in the middle of this, I had a moment of clarity. One morning, it was as if someone had flipped a switch inside me. Despite leaving the hospital unable to walk or eat, I knew I could rebuild my life.

The Power of Support

Throughout this journey, the support of those around me was my lifeline. My mum took over caring for the kids when I couldn't, and I can't even begin to imagine the fear she must have felt. And yet, she was always there, steady, strong and loving. My kids adore her, and so do I.

My husband showed up to every chemotherapy session, doing everything he could to keep our family together. And then there was Natasha, my friend, who came with me to every appointment and helped with the kids when I couldn't.

Nicola from The Wonderful Wig Company knew exactly what I was going through, having been through her cancer journey. Losing my hair was heartbreaking, but she helped me find a wig that became my armour. It was a small thing, but it gave me back a sense of control.

Letting Myself Feel

Through all of this, I learned that allowing myself to feel my emotions wasn't a sign of weakness, but a sign of strength. It was my way of honouring what I was going through. Suppressing my feelings would have only prolonged the pain and stress. By facing my emotions head-on, I was able to heal more fully, both physically and emotionally.

It's okay to be scared. It's okay to feel angry. It's okay to cry. These emotions are valid. The more you let yourself feel them, the more you can move forward. Of course, I still mourn the life I once had. I miss the girl I was before all of this. I cried when I lost my hair, and there are days when I still yearn for my old life. But I've come to accept that this is who I am now. And in many ways, I'm stronger for it. I don't sweat the small stuff anymore, and I cherish every moment with the people I love.

Recently, I achieved a long-held dream by joining a graduate program, which I often thought would never be possible. Despite everything that I have been through, I am making my future a reality. Because here's the truth: The darkness doesn't last forever. You will find your way through it, one step at a time.

30

Reclaiming My Future - My Way

By Carlos Muñez

The day I noticed a lump on the side of my neck, my life shifted in ways I could never have anticipated. Cancer was the last thing I expected to deal with, especially as a young, healthy person with no symptoms other than that lump. When I told my mum about the upcoming scan, we didn't even consider cancer. But after months of inconclusive tests and that final biopsy, I found myself sitting in a room with my mum and a consultant as the words "thyroid cancer" felt like such a shock.

At first, we were reassured, there was a treatment plan, and optimism was encouraged. But how could I face this, on top of everything else? I already struggled with feeling "too much" as a transgender man, too complicated, too burdensome. My instinct was to keep it to myself, even from my girlfriend. I thought about ending our relationship just to spare her the mess of my life. But when I finally opened up, her unwavering support was like lifting a boulder off my chest. For the first time in months, I could breathe, and we started dreaming of the future again.

Still, daily life felt foreign. I pressed pause on college because I couldn't focus, and even simple routines felt overwhelming. I hated the tumour on my neck, hated what it represented. Surgery was the first step, but it wasn't the last. More tests revealed the cancer had spread to the other side of my thyroid and lymph nodes so more surgery, more waiting. My friends' lives moved forward, but mine was stuck in limbo, much like during my gender transition when I had to wait, and hope, while everyone else seemed to move on.

Convincing the team at the Gender Identity Clinic that my health journey wouldn't impede my hormone treatment became an unexpected hurdle. It required a series of exchanged letters between consultants to ensure mutual agreement that my transition could continue. I refused to halt my journey of transitioning just because of my diagnosis.

On the day of surgery, my mum and auntie accompanied me. Sadly, subsequent scans and tests revealed that the cancer had spread to the other side of my thyroid, necessitating its complete removal along with the lymph nodes.

Young Oncology Unit

After surgery came radioiodine therapy, a week-long isolation stint that left me feeling even lonelier. My time at The Christie Hospital was marked by the eerie quiet of isolation, made worse by the chaos of the Manchester riots just outside. When I got home, there were still precautions, separate washing and separating everything to prevent radiation exposure. But I could finally hug my mum again and see my girlfriend.

Then I was referred to the Young Oncology Unit (YOU), a place that became my sanctuary. I met people who understood, *really understood,* what I was going through. Mike and Chris, two of my best mates, were there for me at every turn, and my girlfriend, who had stood by me from day one, helped me stay grounded. My mum had this incredible faith that it would all become just a memory one day. Now, as a parent myself, I can only imagine how scared she must have been while being my source of calm.

I think often of the people I met along the way, those who aren't here anymore. It's a constant reminder to live fully, to embrace every moment and to love deeply.

Lessons That Stick

When I was first diagnosed, I realised pretty quickly that I couldn't control the cancer itself, but I could control how I responded. Finding those little areas where I had agency helped me get through.

I allowed myself the occasional binge day, comfort food and TV marathons were necessary but I also made the effort to eat well, take walks, and stay connected to friends. Simple things that made all the difference.

My girlfriend never let me feel alone, even when I was at my lowest. Saturday nights became sacred for us: Domino's pizza, bad TV, and dreaming about the future. Some people might find it hard to plan beyond the day when faced with cancer, but I found comfort in it. If thinking about the future makes you feel better, then don't hold back. It's okay to hope.

And then there was the power of shared experiences. Meeting others going through similar journeys was incredibly empowering. There's something about being able to say, "Me too," that makes the load feel a little lighter. Talking openly with people who understood shifted the focus from "Why me?" to "How can we get through this together?"

One thing I learned is that finishing treatment doesn't mean the fight is over. The long-term effects, both physical and emotional, are real, and the challenges don't disappear just because you're "cancer-free."

For those of us who survive, there's also the guilt. The feeling that we owe it to those who didn't make it to live fully and without regrets. That's a weight, too, and it's important to take care of yourself in the process.

Building a Future

Strangely, I owe much of my future to two things: my gender transition and my cancer diagnosis. Both taught me resilience, and both showed me my own strength.

After surgeries and treatments, after finding my people and reconnecting with myself, I realised I wasn't just surviving, I was thriving.

I passed my first year of college with distinctions in every module, a far cry from the uncertainty I'd felt at the start. And with my girlfriend, now my wife, by my side, I wasn't going to be left behind. When she started her first year at university, I applied too, and I got in.

It's surreal sometimes, how much has changed. I don't even recognise the person I was before all this, and I'm excited to see who I'll become next. The future, once clouded by fear, now feels wide open.

31

Pride Through Adversity

By Steve Wood

Standing by Nicola's side at Buckingham Palace for the King's garden party was surreal. She was being honoured for her contributions to society, but realistically knowing we were there because she got cancer, was a strange thing to contemplate. I wouldn't wish for anyone to get a diagnosis of cancer, but Nicola has shown me that you can create change in your own life and thousands of others.

It all began with a small lump Nicola noticed on her breast. Like many people who work out regularly, I thought it was nothing serious, maybe an injury or a calcium deposit. When I felt it, I said, "It's probably nothing but best to get it checked out".

Nicola, being Nicola, chose not to follow my advice and waited a few weeks. The lump didn't go away so she eventually went to get checked out. We then had to wait for the results, but neither of us was particularly worried. Nic was pretty blasé about it, and so I took it that it was okay for me to be too.

The doctors told her that there was probably nothing to worry about, that the tiny lump was most likely to be a non-dangerous growth, maybe a cyst. Because of this, I wasn't with Nicola when she was given the news at the hospital. She had mentioned a hospital appointment, but this was very common for Nic as she had her rheumatology consultations at this hospital and always insisted on going to them alone too.

When I walked into the living room after her appointment, time stopped. Nicola was sitting there, shell-shocked. I had expected an easy thumbs-up and be on my way to my physio appointment, which I was already running late for, but from just looking at her, I knew it hadn't gone well. I wanted to stay but Nicola kept shouting at me to go to my appointment, she would be fine! It felt like I was watching the conversation from above and everything was collapsing around us.

I wanted to run away, but instead, I went to physio, feeling stunned. On reflection, not my greatest move to date. That hour was one of the longest of my life. I dreaded going home, knowing or indeed not knowing what was waiting for me and our family. When I returned Nicola was in the same position as when I had left. Her sister Michelle was also there comforting her. They were talking about how to tell their brother Stephen, not wanting to give such terrible news when he'd only just had a baby.

My wife is nothing but pragmatic and was now obsessing not just over her future but also organising mine and Gabriel's lives. I was told sternly by her that if the worst happened, she wanted me to meet someone else. Gabriel needed a mother and I needed to live a full life without her. It was only a few hours after she was told she had cancer, and she was already planning our lives without her.

I wanted the same as anyone else who faces this situation - my loved one to survive, and to get on with the life you've planned together. For both a patient and their partner, your life gets put on hold and you can't breathe once you've had the diagnosis. You are simply waiting to know what's going to happen next unsure of how much your lives are going to be turned upside down.

The Waiting Game

From then on, it felt like we were always waiting. Waiting for surgery, waiting for test results, waiting for the next step in treatment. The uncertainty was overwhelming, and even though we tried to have "cancer-free days," it was hard to escape. Everywhere we looked, there were reminders of cancer – TV ads, movie characters, funeral cars. I gripped the TV remote so I was ready to flick the channel over if anything remotely linked to cancer came on. It felt like we were being haunted by it. But the worst wait by far was that one-year mark, waiting to see if the cancer had come back or if Nicola was still in the clear.

Back in the consultation room for the results, I remember thinking they were going to tell us it was back – I'm not sure if it was a pessimistic thing or just the fact that we were used to hearing bad news. I think Nicola felt this too. Armed for the worst, we went back to the hospital. Neither of us even dared to share what we were thinking and fearing.

We arranged for a babysitter to look after Gabriel so that we could deal with the news we got privately before making a battle plan. We decided that whether it was good or bad news, we would go to the local pub and discuss the next steps. I have never felt as nervous or afraid in my life. I wasn't showing it though as my wife was sitting next to me, and I knew if I showed her how I felt, it would make things ten times worse for her.

As we sat opposite the surgeon who had originally saved Nic's life, I felt like I was going to throw up. He examined Nicola, simply smiled, and said she was one year clear. I was sweating and trying to work out if I'd like his job or despise it. Nicola jumped up, started crying and hugged the surgeon tight; she likes hugging. We then went off to the pub as planned, for more hugging.

Impact on the Family

I couldn't let my guard down. My job was to protect my family, and that meant keeping everything negative at bay. I got angry at anyone who brought up cancer to Nicola, but I also got mad if they acted like it wasn't happening. You were better to stay out of my way. It felt like every conversation, every moment, was tied to this diagnosis. Looking back my anger was the only way I knew how to express my sadness and grief.

Telling our son Gabriel was heart-wrenching. He was so young and didn't understand what was going on, however, kids are quite perceptive. We had to be honest with him, even though I didn't know for sure I was telling him the truth – that mammy was poorly but she was going to be okay.

When the Fire Returns

One day, after a particularly tough session of radiotherapy, Nicola saw a sign about hair loss in the hospital. Half-jokingly, I told her she could help women who were losing their hair. She didn't hear me at the time, but a few days later, something clicked. Nicola found her fire again. She dove headfirst into researching how to support women with hair loss, and a new business idea was born.

That moment brought my wife back to life. It gave her a sense of purpose and, in a way, helped her heal emotionally. This wasn't just work for Nicola, it was therapy. Helping others through their cancer journeys helped her process her own, and in the process, she's changed the hair loss industry in ways that are deeply personal and transformative.

She wanted to provide a service where it was more personable and not a conveyor belt giving out hair in boxes for sick people. It was all she talked about, but I thought, at least she's not obsessing about cancer. After what she'd been through, it worried me that it might negatively affect her mental health being in such close contact with people battling cancer who were so sick, and often end of life. This worried me - remember my protector mode?

Moving Forward with Pride

Nicola's speeches and work have impacted countless lives, and it's incredible to see how much she's achieved. I am proud beyond words, not just of her strength through cancer, but of her ability to take one of the darkest experiences of our lives and turn it into something that helps others. Watching her comfort other women, knowing exactly what they're going through, makes everything we've been through feel like it had a purpose.

I am so proud of what my wife has dealt with and how she is helping and guiding other people through their cancers. Cancer may have thrown our lives into chaos, but Nicola took that chaos and created something incredible.

32

Boldly Living

By Nell Wright

Cancer didn't just throw a spanner in my plans, it put my entire life on pause. I had to skip two girls' holidays, miss out on family trips, stop going to college, and cancel my first holiday with my boyfriend. Yet even as cancer tried to rob me of all these moments, I made a choice: cancer could only take what I allowed it to, and I wasn't going to let it take everything.

When I finally got my diagnosis, six months after getting sick, I didn't react much. While my parents were breaking down, I sat there, strangely unfazed. Maybe it was my way of silently declaring that cancer wasn't going to define my life.

Navigating the Rollercoaster

My first stint with chemo lasted four months through a port. But then the cancer came back, stronger. This time, it was chemo through a Hickman line, followed by a stem cell transplant. Remission came, but not for long, within four months, I relapsed. My Stage 2 cancer had escalated to Stage 4, and with it came more chemo, immunotherapy, and another transplant, this time from a donor.

Through it all, my boyfriend stayed by my side. We'd only been together for six months when I was diagnosed, and now it's been two and a half years. The journey hasn't just changed me, it's changed our relationship, too. I was also referred to a psychologist to support me, and I began seeing them weekly.

Refusing to Sit Still

Even as I lost my hair, I refused to lose myself. I experimented with wigs, trying different colours and styles. I learned to glue lace fronts down like a pro. Some people didn't love my choices, but I didn't care. You wouldn't walk up to someone and criticise their real hair, so why do people think it's okay just because it's a wig? For me, this was about confidence and I wasn't going to let anyone take that from me.

I lost my hair and looked different, but I wasn't going to let that stop me from living. I went out, I partied, I had fun. And yes, people were surprised by how much I went out for a cancer patient, but here's the thing: Not all cancer stories fit the stereotype of frailty. Just because you're sick doesn't mean you can't live. I embraced every moment, whether it was a night out at the club or attending a festival.

Own Your Health, Own Your Life

Of course, it wasn't all carefree nights out. I stayed informed. I knew my symptoms, what to watch out for, and who to call if anything went wrong. The key was finding a balance and living boldly, but also staying vigilant about my health.

Cancer delayed my education and pushed back my start at university, and that stung me. But after wallowing for a bit, I realised that dwelling on what I couldn't control wasn't going to help. So, I focused on what I *could* control: making the most of the time I had. I made a promise to myself that I wouldn't waste a moment waiting for the storm to pass. If I had the strength to live, I would.

Humour as a Lifeline

Humour became my armour. I cracked jokes about my hair – if someone had a bad haircut, I'd tease them, saying

I preferred mine. I wasn't afraid to laugh, even at cancer. Laughter made it bearable. I even used my wig as a trump card to get into places I technically shouldn't have, pulling it off for a laugh when bouncers questioned my age. Maybe it wasn't polite, but it was a tool, and I wasn't afraid to use it. I never hesitated to play the cancer card.

Prioritise You

If there's one thing I've learned through all of this, it's to take care of yourself, physically and mentally. And that doesn't look the same for everyone. Maybe your "self-care" is binge-watching Netflix or hitting the gym, maybe it's dancing all night long or taking quiet walks. Whatever it is, it's valid. You get to define it. Cancer tried to stop me from living, but I refused to let it dictate my terms.

33

Space and Support

By Kathryn Turner

Receiving my diagnosis was one of the hardest moments in my breast cancer journey. The two-week wait between seeing my GP and my appointment at the breast clinic was agonising. Somehow, I knew it was cancer. Despite trying to prepare my husband (who had already lost his mother to breast cancer) and my parents, they all reassured me it was just a cyst. But I knew better. The night before the appointment, I couldn't stop shaking, my body consumed by fear.

At the clinic, my husband wasn't allowed in. After the mammogram and ultrasound, the confirmation came: breast cancer. I barely remember the nurse asking if I had anyone to take me home; I just told her my husband was waiting in the car. Walking out to him, my legs felt like jelly. When he asked, "What is it?" all I could manage was, "It's what I thought it was."

Breaking the news to our parents, family, and especially our children, aged 16, 14, and 5, was the toughest part. I hadn't even had the space to process it myself. How could I prepare my kids for something that still felt surreal to me?

Facing the Hardest Truths

The news hit me like a ton of bricks, Grade 3 breast cancer. I couldn't help but panic, fearing I had limited time left. The overwhelming emotions of frustration, anger, and even guilt despite living a healthy life, started to take over. We discussed what we were going to say to my parents, family, and children. This was difficult, without the time and space to digest the diagnosis before worrying about everyone else and the feeling of "letting people down" by having cancer.

I dreaded telling my children. I reassured them that it was curable with treatment, but deep down, I had my fears. I wondered if I should create memory boxes for them. I remember thinking, "Would my boys manage without me? Would my little girl even remember me?"

Navigating Treatment

Chemotherapy was the first step in my treatment, followed by surgery and radiotherapy. The chemo was horrendous, I felt sick, ached all over and lost my hair. The lumpectomy was physically easier by comparison. I'd never slept so deeply as I did during that operation, not since my diagnosis. The radiotherapy, though not painful, drained my energy, leaving me utterly exhausted.

I had eight cycles of chemo, one every three weeks. Each session felt like climbing a mountain, but I focused on milestones. When I finally rang that bell after my last session, it was just me, my husband, and the nurses who had cared for me, quiet, emotional, and deeply personal.

Accepting Support

During treatment, I stuck to the advice I was given, limiting contact, staying home, eating healthily and getting as much rest as possible. I accepted the help of my family, especially my parents. They visited daily, helped with school pick-ups and brought me homemade soup. On the hardest days of each infusion cycle, they took my daughter to their house to shield her from how unwell I looked.

I missed out on a lot: my son's prom, school events, even birthday parties I'd organised but couldn't attend. Having the loving support of my family made me aware that if anything happened to me, my children would be cared for and this brought immense comfort.

Finding Strength in Laughter

Losing my hair was hard, but what hit me most was losing my eyebrows and lashes. It was a constant reminder every time I saw my face. Attending an online session of Look Good, Feel Good helped a bit; they even sent me makeup freebies, which lifted my spirits.

As much as I could, I tried to find humour in my situation. My little girl was upset at first when my hair fell out, but eventually, we all found moments to laugh about it. I stopped fixating on the mirror and eventually embraced my baldness. I even found comfort in my wig and caps, which became a part of my new normal.

The Power of Perspective

Over time, I learned to take things one step at a time. Each new stage of my diagnosis felt overwhelming at first, but when broken down, it became manageable. There were surprises along the way, like learning I was "node-positive" after initially being told I was "node-negative," but I adapted.

I've come to realise how much support matters and how essential it is to lean into the relationships that lift you. Sometimes, it's better when people don't try to fill the silence with words. Instead of endlessly searching online for answers, I've shifted to reading things that help me get through each day, like dietary tips that genuinely benefit my treatment.

After much thought, I chose a synthetic wig similar in length to my pre-diagnosis hair, but lighter with a fringe for a change. I didn't wear it at home due to the heat, but when I did go out, especially after treatment, I was pleased with it. I opted for synthetic over real hair for its low maintenance. I also bought plain chemo caps, which were useful and comfortable, and a bed cap for sleeping.

I would recommend a silk pillowcase as it is soft and cool on your face to sleep on. I accepted the prospect of losing my hair quite early on and although it was upsetting and shocking at first, it's amazing how quickly you get used to it. I found that I stopped looking or noticing it in the mirror. Being bald almost became insignificant in the scheme of things.

I've had the expected comments about my hair like, "I didn't recognise you there" or when I returned to work,

"Your hair is really short" or when I went to a kid's party post-treatment, "Are you Millie's mam, we haven't met before" from someone whom I have spoken to loads of times. I've learnt to let these wash over me.

Moving Forward with Gratitude

Since my diagnosis, my perspective has shifted in profound ways. I've learned to appreciate the little things - walking my child to school, reading them a bedtime story or cooking a meal for my family. It's easy to take health for granted until it's suddenly in question. Now, I don't let the small worries get to me as they used to. Life's simple pleasures feel like gifts, and I embrace them with a newfound sense of gratitude.

Create distractions - I had lots of treats! My parents kindly bought me a Kindle and I started reading a lot. I accepted a slower pace of life than what I was used to, and I focused on getting better.

I met some amazing and inspirational people who I am still close to today. Getting to spend more time with parents was a bonus too as I was unable to work.

Focus on one step at a time. When you are given your diagnosis and treatment plan it sounds overwhelming and not doable but if you just focus on one stage at a time and break it down into manageable pieces it helps mentally. Instead of constantly searching online for outcomes, focus on reading helpful resources that can assist with your treatment, such as books on beneficial dietary tips.

When supporting others, offer advice and guidance when asked, but be mindful not to impose yourself on their journey, as everyone's experience is unique. Self-resilience is crucial, and it's essential not to compare.

34

One Day at a Time

By Emma Ogle

I often meet our teenage inpatients and their families a few days after they hear the words "It's cancer." They may have come from different hospitals and wards and landed with us here in the Teenage Cancer Unit in the Great North Children's Hospital.

You can't quite comprehend how they are feeling, everyone reacts in their own way. I try to be a friendly face to our teenagers and their loved ones, so they know there's someone here who isn't medical, who isn't trying to give them some news or results, and someone they can find if they just want to have a chat or need a distraction.

I've had some meaningful conversations with parents in the kitchen while making a cuppa. Here they have space outside the cubicle away from their loved one, to say how it is in that moment for them. We can talk about all sorts; work, family, dogs, treatment, worry, friends, hair loss and coping. I let them choose what they want to let off their chest. By engaging in conversations about everyday topics, it creates a sense of normality for them. This simple act makes the overwhelming situation feel more manageable.

The same goes for when I do activities with teenagers. Any topic of conversation comes up; "What's the latest watch on Netflix? What's on your "for you" page on TikTok? What do you like doing in your spare time?" The conversations are important. They serve as a distraction away from cancer, treatment and side effects, allowing them not only to take it day by day but also to find comfort in the most mundane of activities, which goes a long way.

This is our patient's chance for them to tell me who they are, away from the hospital bed and their diagnosis. That might look like sitting next to each other, saying very little, playing Mario Kart on the big screen. Very rarely does anyone beat a teenager on a video game! Active treatment makes our young people tired, sick and lethargic; each day is different for them.

Embracing Daily Struggles

Adolescents experiment with identity and push boundaries, they are no longer children, but not yet adults. When teenage patients are told their treatment may cause hair loss, this is a huge blow for them. Their hair is their identity, as are eyebrows and lashes. They don't want to be different from their peers. There are many tears shed over hair loss on this ward, and I always want patients and families to know it's okay to feel that way. Our girls are always interested in wigs and it's a pleasure to offer them a real hair wig through Little Princess Trust, as well as an NHS voucher for synthetic wigs.

We maintain a wig board on the ward, showcasing photos of our teenagers both with and without their wigs. It's a reassuring sight for them, helping them realise they're not alone in their journey. Each glance offers a little more comfort and confidence, as they grow accustomed to their appearance without hair, one day at a time.

I help some patients with cutting or shaving their hair if that's their wish. I leave it to them to decide but try and advise if it starts getting uncomfortable. Once they see lots of strands on their pillow, they prefer to just shave it off. It takes two to three weeks after a referral to the Little Princess Trust to get a real hair wig. The wigs I have seen over the years have gotten better and better, sometimes it's hard to tell if it is a wig!

Our patients take pride in their wigs and start feeling like themselves when they get home and can put their makeup and wig on to go out! I have also seen many teenagers who rock the bald look, sporting an array of hats, scarves and beanies, embracing their changing appearance with resilience.

It's always uplifting to encounter teenagers on the outpatient ward and across social platforms. Learning about their recent activities, whether returning to school or enjoying time with friends, is truly heartening. Engaging in social interactions consistently boosts their spirits.

As their hair begins to grow back and their eyebrows and lashes regain thickness, a subtle transformation unfolds. You can detect a newfound sparkle in their eyes, reflecting a growing sense of vitality and hope with each passing day.

My Advice for Teenagers with Cancer

During difficult times I hear myself say, "Take one day at a time." This simple yet genuine piece of advice sums up the importance of living in the moment, urging patients to focus solely on the present without allowing worries about the future to overwhelm them. For teenagers grappling with the challenges of cancer, this mindset can serve as a lifeline, offering solace and strength in the face of uncertainty.

Rediscovering motivation beyond treatment can be challenging for teenagers. Their lives may feel like they've been upended, with peers moving on and energy levels diminished. Starting with small steps, such as taking a walk with a friend, assisting with meal preparation, or hosting a movie night, can reignite their interests and restore their self-assurance. Again, it's in everyday activities that they can build their confidence.

I always extend an invitation to our peer support social meetups, where we create a welcoming environment for teens to connect and engage in enjoyable activities like bowling or crazy golf – with plenty of food, of course!

Bringing a friend along to the first few socials can ease any nerves about attending alone. We organise trips throughout the year, including the highly anticipated sailing excursion with the Ellen MacArthur Cancer Trust to Scotland. Participants have the opportunity to sail, bond with peers and create lasting memories.

One touching moment that stands out is when a teenage patient shared her experience of attending prom. She recounted how she enjoyed the day, seamlessly juggling her preparations. She even dropped off her wig at the salon for styling while getting her nails done, a thoughtful gesture that saved her precious time.

These are the moments that strike me the most: when patients, despite facing the weight of their diagnoses, manage to uncover a glimmer of hope, using it to brighten their daily lives. It's these instances of resilience and determination that truly touch my heart and fuel my dedication to continue supporting them in any way I can.

Reflections from Nicola

Cancer doesn't come with a manual, but it definitely comes with a roller coaster of feelings, so buckle up, let those tears flow when needed, and don't forget to throw in some laughter for good measure. Embracing every emotion is a vital step toward healing, and it's okay if that means crying into a tub of ice cream some days! When life throws curveballs, whether it's a diagnosis or identity struggles, reclaiming your future means daring to dream again. After all, hope is the fertiliser that makes life bloom, even if you sometimes feel like you're knee-deep in the weeds.

True pride comes from facing life's darkest moments with resilience, love and an unwavering commitment to family. There's nothing quite like realising you've been through the worst and still have the strength to smile, support and keep going. Cancer might make you feel like life's been put on hold, but that doesn't mean you can't still turn up the volume, put on your favourite outfit (or wig), and hit the dance floor. Whether it's a festival, a holiday, or just a cheeky night out with friends, remember: cancer doesn't take away your right to live fully.

Whether it's family, friends or that one person who knows exactly how to make you laugh at the worst moments, it's all about balance. Remember, saying "no" to others sometimes means saying "yes" to your well-being. Focusing on each day, rather than letting the future overwhelm you, is an act of self-care. Some days will feel heavy, but taking things moment by moment keeps the weight manageable. The collective journey through cancer, as reflected in these stories, is a testament to the incredible resilience of the human spirit. Each person has faced unimaginable challenges, from the fear of diagnosis to the emotional rollercoaster of treatment, yet they've found strength in their vulnerability. Whether through embracing their emotions, finding joy amid adversity or holding on to dreams for the future, these stories highlight the power of hope, humour and human connection.

Conclusion
The End is Simply
the Beginning

My nana used to tell me that people were born with two ears and one mouth for a reason. There's a similar expression I learned at the hospice where I volunteer to do hair, "Listening is not the same as waiting to speak." When you truly listen to someone, you hear every word, every fear and every piece of hope. Sometimes, when people talk about their cancer, they don't need advice, solutions or comparisons. Often, the simple act of saying, "I've got cancer," is hard enough.

A wise nurse once told me that when you don't know what to say, it's okay to say exactly that, "I'm sorry, I don't know what to say." That's it. That's enough. Full stop. Listening, really listening, can mean more than any words.

As you've read through the stories in this book, I hope you've truly heard the voices of those who've shared their journeys. Their stories of strength, resilience and survival offer something valuable: a reminder that you're not alone and that your story is still yours to write. It can feel like everything about your day is different and you become a puppet, with the hospital being your master, pulling your strings. Cancer can change your life, but it doesn't have to define it.

In some of my darkest moments, I felt like I was only "Nicola with cancer." It seemed as if my whole identity was replaced with that diagnosis. I believed cancer had stolen everything: my future, my health, my career, my choices. But as you've read, I learned that while cancer takes, it also gives. It shifts your perspective and challenges you to find new ways to live and thrive.

Cancer amplified my emotions to the point where I let them consume me. On certain days, I took everything to heart immediately. If someone was late, I assumed it was intentional. If someone glanced at me in the supermarket, I was sure they were judging my weight gain. And if I dared to think about the future, it felt like staring into a black hole of despair. I became short-tempered and snappy, often without realising it, because I was carrying so much unhappiness. It took time, but I eventually learned to step back and give myself space, allowing me to respond thoughtfully rather than react with raw emotion. Not letting cancer define every part of my thinking helped me regain control over how I dealt with situations.

Progress isn't linear, and on the hardest days, I invite you to open this book and remind yourself that you are not alone, and more importantly, that you are not your cancer. You're still you, and while cancer may be part of your journey, it doesn't have to consume your every thought or conversation. A coach once told me, "The more attention you give something, the more it grows." Don't let cancer become your whole life.

A Vision Realised

What started as a personal journey through cancer has blossomed into something much bigger, The Wonderful Wig Company. Born from a simple desire to help women feel beautiful during one of the most difficult times in their lives, this company now employs over 20 people across 10 sites in the UK and has supported over 15,000 women. In addition to providing wigs, we've expanded into charity work and free training for salon professionals, breaking down the barriers for those facing hair loss.

Initially, we started with Sunderland Hospital, but soon after witnessing the impact we made, I wanted to help more hospitals in the Northeast. I worked tirelessly to secure contracts with almost every hospital in the region and earned a place on the NHS framework, which allowed us to expand even further.

One of our biggest goals is to integrate hair loss services into regular salons, making it possible for women to continue seeing their usual hairdresser even after losing their hair. This goal has driven us to partner with salons across the country, offering training programs to ensure that every town has a place where people facing hair loss can feel comfortable and supported. Through this initiative, we're transforming the way hair loss is handled in the beauty industry.

Can you imagine a better scenario than that? Just being able to go to your regular hairdresser is great. You feel comfortable there. She knows you inside out and already loves you. That's what should happen when you lose your hair.

I've recently set up a not-for-profit charity called the Inclusion Hair Network, which helps create safe, skilled, and understanding salons across the country for minority and LGBTQIA+ people. The CIC aims to ensure that anyone from any community can feel confident stepping into hair, beauty and hair loss salons.

My Journey of Resilience

While The Wonderful Wig Company has been a huge professional accomplishment, my personal journey has been equally transformative. Overcoming invasive breast cancer wasn't just a battle against illness, it was a test of endurance, mental strength and emotional resilience. Alongside my health challenges, I have been an advocate, a mother, a wife and a voice for those going through similar struggles. My keynote speeches have shared the lessons I've learned, focusing on gratitude and growth, even in the face of adversity.

As a mother, I've been deeply committed to ensuring my son, Gabriel, sees that resilience is not about never falling, but about always getting back up. I've been open with him about my journey, teaching him the value of emotional response over reaction, and the importance of kindness to oneself.

Through cancer, I discovered new strengths. I transformed my pain into a mission to help others, founding The Wonderful Wig Company and working every day to make a difference in the lives of those affected by cancer. This journey has shaped me into a woman more alive and purposeful than ever before, and I'm grateful for each new day.

My mission now is to be heard and understood, and to continue making an impact, one story, one wig, and one person at a time.

Another thing I learned throughout my journey, and that I'm constantly reminding my son Gabriel about, is that it is better to respond rather than react. It's so easy to take things personally when you have cancer. Slowing down and assessing if your reaction is more about how you are feeling rather than what the person is saying, is useful. In the same way, you listen and not simply wait your turn to speak, you can take the time and space to absorb all the things that are happening to you and around you before responding to them from an objective viewpoint.

Since cancer, I actively do things that scare the sh*t out of me. On the other side of scary things is living, real living. I applied for and was selected to deliver a TEDx Talk. This was a powerful moment of validation, proof that I had not only survived but was thriving. Standing on that iconic red dot, I felt the weight of the moment, knowing that in just 12 minutes, I had the chance to reach people around the world with my message about hair loss and its deeper implications. It wasn't just about cosmetics or vanity.

I wanted to highlight the profound emotional and psychological effects of losing one's hair, something I'd experienced firsthand as a hairdresser who became a patient. I spoke about self-esteem, confidence and mental health, showing how hair loss can alter a person's identity in ways many don't realise.

The talk was a vulnerable moment for me, especially given my journey from the radiotherapy dots to the TED stage red dot. But it was also a triumphant one, filled with purpose and a determination to change perceptions. This was another opportunity to scream from the rooftops how important hair loss is and pushed me so far out of my comfort zone.

Beyond the Diagnosis

In one of my keynotes, I shared all the reasons I've come to feel grateful for my cancer journey. You can access it through the resources by scanning this QR code:

My goal in sharing this story was to help others see that, like me, they can use their experience as fuel to transform pain into something meaningful, even beautiful. This fight continues, and it's one we can all be a part of.

I'm not taking my life for granted, and I don't want you to either. There is life during cancer, and for most there is life after it. You get to choose what they both look like.

If these stories have touched you, and you're inspired to continue spreading hope to others, I'd love to stay connected. Visit me at www.iamnicolawood.com and let's keep this journey going together. If this book has helped you feel a little less like an outsider in this club no one asked to join, then I know I've done my job.

Epilogue

One of the key insights that emerges from all the stories in this book is that receiving the "all clear" is far from the end of the journey. Ringing the bell to signify the completion of treatment is not the final chapter but rather the beginning of a new and equally challenging phase. Life after cancer continues to demand just as much mental and emotional resilience as the physical battle did. The recovery process includes coping with ongoing medical checkups, emotional highs and lows and the fear of recurrence, which can be just as taxing as the treatment itself.

As I prepare to wrap up this book for publication, the timing is poignant – I'm approaching my eight-year checkup. To give you a glimpse of what life looks like many years after diagnosis and treatment, I've documented 24 hours of my life. It highlights how, even years later, the experience continues to shape everyday life.

Eight Years After My Breast Cancer Diagnosis

Sunday

Today was all about self-care, something I never prioritised before cancer. I woke up hangover-free (a big change from earlier in my life) and met a friend for coffee and exercise at the beach. Staying active helps keep my arthritis in check and I am much more mindful of my long-term health now. After a healthy breakfast, I indulged in an afternoon nap, knowing that taking care of myself was key, especially the day before my annual scan.

Sunday Evening

As I head to bed on the eve of my annual breast clinic scans, I'm aware that I'm at the point of bringing this book to a close. Each year, the worry lessens a bit, similar to grieving a loss - it never fully goes away, but it affects me less over time. I'm grateful I get to check that I am still clear, rather than seeing how much it has progressed. I didn't want to burden my family with my worries, so I offered up a prayer to express everything on my mind.

I'm sitting in bed, struggling with the "What ifs." My mind keeps returning to this book - what if I have to write another chapter titled "The Cancer is Back"? I grabbed a pen and paper to jot down my thoughts, feelings and emotions. Then, I started listing all the reasons I'm grateful for cancer. I even chuckled, realising this could be a book in itself: *All the Reasons I'm Grateful for Cancer.*

- I now understand I don't need to be Superwoman all the time.

- I am grateful for my friends who can make me laugh, even on my darkest of days.

- Cancer pushed me to make major lifestyle changes - now I am fitter, healthier and stronger.

- Every day, I wake up with a purpose: to change an outdated system, support those dealing with hair loss and impact the future of hair care.

- I also get to bring this book to life, filled with heartfelt stories that give people a voice.

- I'm grateful for my incredible husband, wonderful son and siblings, who have been by my side through it all.

Check out the resources at the start of this book to see more of my gratitudes and how to join our social media campaign, Why I am Grateful for Cancer.

Monday 5am

I woke up before my alarm, with the weight of my appointment on my mind. I headed downstairs and opened my pill box, which holds a mix of supplements for my hair, skin, and nails, along with Vitamin D, Tamoxifen, and injection for my arthritis. This daily routine is a constant reminder that I'm still working to prevent cancer. Tamoxifen, the medication that blocks my oestrogen and keeps me in medical menopause, is known for causing many side effects. Even eight years on, it's a reminder that the journey is never truly over.

Exercise helped me cope this morning and I kept busy – definitely a strategy I rely on when facing things, I'd rather avoid.

Harry Potter strikes again as I batch cook for the next three months and run from room to room, sorting, folding, lifting and moving things – just like I did eight years ago when I was awaiting appointments and results.

It feels different now. I've changed, inside and out. My body is stronger, healthier, and slimmer. I've trained my body to be more capable than it was eight years ago. I've gained clarity, resilience, and acceptance over the last eight years.

Monday Mid-Morning

I get a message from a friend of my sister-in-law's via Messenger. Her friend, recently diagnosed with cancer at 30, is terrified of losing her hair and doesn't know anyone else who has been through this. She reached out to me for help, knowing I could support her. Instinctively, I wanted to call her right away – I know I can offer guidance. But then I realised I already have a lot on my plate today. I get these kinds of messages often and have to remind myself that I need to prioritise my well-being first. If I don't, I won't be able to give my best support. While this situation is exactly why I do what I do, I decided I couldn't help her today. She'll be the first on my list tomorrow. It is okay to say "No" and "Not right now."

Monday at the Hospital

As I'm wandering through the corridors looking for the purple zone, I am reminded of every single time I have been here before. I hate the purple zone. Even though I know it will be fine and I'm here for a check-up and I get to see all of the incredible nurses and staff – it fills me with dread.

Monday in the Waiting Room

Sitting in the waiting room, wearing the gown, brought me back to the early days. I'm no longer blasé – it feels different now. I don't want to take it for granted. I've done countless self-checks to prepare, knowing this day was coming. If I could spot any changes, it wouldn't be a surprise when they examined me.

I've spent time looking at my chest, and noticing how different it is now. I am grateful that I have breasts. I am grateful regardless of how they look. I am in total acceptance, knowing they look different and feel different, and that doesn't make it bad or wrong.

I don't enjoy being back here, surrounded by other women – old, young, with partners, without partners and knowing that statistically some of them are going to get bad news and some of them are here to celebrate getting the all clear, others are here for prevention and screening. It is surreal when you've been through it to sit on the other side knowing what awaits in that room.

Monday in the Examination Room

Today involves blood tests, a mammogram, a physical examination, and another appointment for an MRI.

Monday in the Car

The tests are done, and now I am waiting for the MRI and results. It's a relief to be finished but the nurse mentioned that when I turn 50, my screening will become less frequent. While that's a positive, it also feels unsettling, as regular check-ups have been a safety net.

I'm relieved, but I know the waiting game is never easy.

As much as I appreciate seeing everyone at the hospital, it's a reminder of where it all began.

Monday Afternoon

I'm having a little wobble. "F*ck. What if I get results in the week and it is back? Do what works, Nicola, go and do some breathing, go and distract yourself," I tell myself. The "What ifs" buzz around in my mind, but I try to ground myself, reminding myself that if a thought starts with "What if," it is probably bullsh*t.

A little later, while trying to keep busy, I accidentally fell down the stairs. It wasn't too bad of an accident, but I did note the irony of me injuring myself today when I was worrying about the future. It reminded me of something Steve once asked Karen at Maggie's in Newcastle, "How do we know if Nicola is cured?" Her reply, "When she dies of something else," made perfect sense then, and still does now. Karen, often referred to in our house as the Oracle of cancer and treatment, has a remarkable ability to explain things in a way that is easy to understand. Steve had been overwhelmed by information during our many appointments, but in just 30 minutes with Karen, everything finally became clear. I laugh to myself, thinking "Good news today, I'm not dying from cancer but from falling down the stairs."

Monday Late Afternoon

I went to the shop to pick up some 50th birthday cards for two friends and smiled to myself. Getting older feels like such a privilege now. Cancer made me appreciate every year, and I welcome each birthday as a pleasure, not something to dread. Bring it on!

Monday Evening

I pick up my journal and allow all my thoughts to spill onto the pages. It's been an emotional day. I've tried to hold it together so my family doesn't feel like they have to rally around me. I don't like the fuss. These moments to write saved my sanity eight years ago and it's become a habit I love and need to contain my wobbles. I'm overcome with gratitude that I'm still here, despite a run-in with the stairs. I get to watch Gabe grow into a man with Steve by my side as we weather the inevitable storms of life together. Who knows what the next eight years will bring?

About the Author

Nicola Wood is a devoted wife, loving mum and cancer advocate who turned her personal journey with invasive breast cancer into a mission to uplift and empower others facing similar challenges.

After receiving her diagnosis at age 36, she underwent treatment and realised that the then-existing hair-loss solutions were outdated and insufficient. This insight inspired her to create a truly bespoke hair-loss service that caters to everyone and everybody – because hair is so incredibly individual.

In 2016, Nicola founded The Wonderful Wig Company, a unique and compassionate service that has so far supported over 15,000 adults and more than 2,000 children experiencing medical hair loss, including those undergoing chemotherapy or living with alopecia.

In 2024, Nicola delivered her first TEDx talk, titled *"Why It's Not Just Hair."* Watched by over 32,000, Nicola shares how hair represents more than just appearance – it embodies self-worth, resilience and a personal journey of healing. She challenges the misconception that hair is about vanity, revealing its profound role in shaping a person's identity.

Nicola's dedication to others has earned her numerous accolades, including Disrupter for Good at the Northern Power Women in 2024, Most Inspiring Businesswoman at the Best Businesswomen Awards in 2023, Health & Beauty Entrepreneur of the Year at the Great British Entrepreneur Awards in 2022 and Most Inspiring Female at the Chamber of Commerce Business Awards in 2021.

Nicola's story is one of resilience, compassion, and transformation – a wife and mother who used her experience to empower and lift others through her work, giving voice and dignity to those facing cancer.

If you'd like to know more about The Wonderful Wig Company, visit their website at wonderfulwigs.co.uk/